M

M

MW00695423

Brent S. E. Rich MD, ATC CAQSM
Director, Utah Valley Sports Medicine
Fellowship Director, Intermountain Healthcare Utah Valley
Sports Medicine Fellowship
Team Physician, Brigham Young University
Head Team Physician, Utah Flash
Team Physician, Utah Valley University

Mitchell K. Pratte, DO, CAQSM
Head Team Physician, Brigham Young University
Associate Fellowship Director, Intermountain Healthcare Utah Valley
Sports Medicine Fellowship

JONES AND BARTLETT PUBLISHERS
Sudbury, Massachusetts
BOSTON   TORONTO   LONDON   SINGAPORE

World Headquarters
Jones and Bartlett Publishers
40 Tall Pine Drive
Sudbury, MA 01776
978-443-5000
info@jbpub.com
www.jbpub.com

Jones and Bartlett Publishers Canada
6339 Ormindale Way
Mississauga, Ontario L5V 1J2
Canada

Jones and Bartlett Publishers International
Barb House, Barb Mews
London W6 7PA
United Kingdom

Jones and Bartlett's books and products are available through most bookstores and online booksellers. To contact Jones and Bartlett Publishers directly, call 800-832-0034, fax 978-443-8000, or visit our website www.jbpub.com.

Substantial discounts on bulk quantities of Jones and Bartlett's publications are available to corporations, professional associations, and other qualified organizations. For details and specific discount information, contact the special sales department at Jones and Bartlett via the above contact information or send an email to specialsales@jbpub.com.

The authors, editor, and publisher have made every effort to provide accurate information. However, they are not responsible for errors, omissions, or for any outcomes related to the use of the contents of this book and take no responsibility for the use of the products and procedures described. Treatments and side effects described in this book may not be applicable to all people; likewise, some people may require a dose or experience a side effect that is not described herein. Drugs and medical devices are discussed that may have limited availability controlled by the Food and Drug Administration (FDA) for use only in a research study or clinical trial. Research, clinical practice, and government regulations often change the accepted standard in this field. When consideration is being given to use of any drug in the clinical setting, the health care provider or reader is responsible for determining FDA status of the drug, reading the package insert, and reviewing prescribing information for the most up-to-date recommendations on dose, precautions, and contraindications, and determining the appropriate usage for the product. This is especially important in the case of drugs that are new or seldom used.

Production Credits
Chief Executive Officer: Clayton Jones
Chief Operating Officer: Don W. Jones, Jr.
President, Higher Education and Professional Publishing: Robert W. Holland, Jr.
V.P., Sales: William J. Kane
V.P., Design and Production: Anne Spencer
V.P., Manufacturing and Inventory Control: Therese Connell
Publisher: Christopher Davis
Senior Acquisitions Editor: Nancy Anastasi Duffy
Senior Editorial Assistant: Jessica Acox
Production Assistant: Ashlee Hazeltine
Marketing Manager: Ilana Goddess
Composition: Newgen
Cover Design: Kristin E. Parker
Cover Image: Reproduced from Andreas Vesalius. *De corporis humani fabrica libri septem.*
  Army Medical Library, 2005. Photo courtesy of National Library of Medicine.
Printing and Binding: Cenveo
Cover Printing: Cenveo

Library of Congress Cataloging-in-Publication Data
Rich, Brent S. E.
  Tarascon sports medicine pocketbook / Brent S.E. Rich, Mitchell K. Pratte.
    p. ; cm.
  title: Sports medicine pocketbook
  Includes index.
  ISBN-13: 978-0-7637-6679-5 (pbk.)
  ISBN-10: 0-7637-6679-8 (pbk.)
  1. Sports medicine--Handbooks, manuals, etc. I. Pratte, Mitchell K. II. Title. III. Title: Sports
medicine pocketbook.
  [DNLM: 1. Sports Medicine--Handbooks. 2. Athletic Injuries--Handbooks. QT 29 R498t
2010]
  RC1211.R53 2010
  617.1'027--dc22
                                        2008053291

6048
Printed in the United States of America
13 12 11 10   10 9 8 7 6 5 4 3 2

DEDICATION

Special thanks to our families for their patience, tolerance, and love.

Lori, Katie, KC, Kristy, and Cougar Rich
and
Lareen, Bethany, Seth, Christiane, Maile, Levi Pratte

CONTENTS

Editorial Board and Contributing Authors

PREFACE

The *Tarascon Sports Medicine Pocketbook* was written as an easy reference guide for Primary Care Sports Medicine providers, residents, and medical students, as well as physical therapists and athletic trainers. The intent was to create a comprehensive one-source pocketbook to outline the common injuries and illnesses that will present in the athletic population. It is not intended to be a detailed reference.

The chapters provide the scaffolding for education of our sports medicine fellows at Utah Valley Sports Medicine. We share this material with prospective fellows, residents, and medical and premed students that rotate in our facility. Over time, these lectures have become more formalized and we thus decided to compile them in book form. We hope this book helps others in understanding musculoskeletal and medical issues in today's sports medicine environment.

Brent S.E. Rich MD, ATC CAQSM
Mitchell K. Pratt DO, CAQSM

ACKNOWLEDGMENTS

Thanks to the Primary Care Sports Medicine Fellows of Utah Valley Sports Medicine: Ben Betteridge, MD, Spencer Richards, MD, Martin Baur, MD, Carol Wilder, MD, Christian Millward, MD, David Cassat, MD, Matt Evans, MD, and Jim Ngatuvai, MD; the athletic training staffs and athletic departments of Brigham Young University and Utah Valley University; and Kirt Kimball, MD, Wayne Mortenson, MD, and Jeff Smith, MD, and Intermountain Health Care.

APPRECIATION

Sincere appreciation to Meredith Church for her assistance in the compilation of this manuscript.

ABBREVIATIONS

AC — acromioclavicular
ACL — anterior cruciate ligament
ACOG — American College of Obstetricians and Gynecologists
AED — automated external defibrillator
AIDS — acquired immunodeficiency syndrome
AFO — ankle–foot orthoses
AP — anterior/posterior (x-ray)
APL — adductor/abductor pollicis longus
ATC — certified athletic trainer
BCAA — branched chain amino acids
BMD — bone mineral density
BMI — body mass index
BMP — basic metabolic profile
BP — blood pressure
BPM — beats per minute
CF — cystic fibrosis
CO — cardiac output
CSF — cerebrospinal fluid
CT — computed tomography
CXR — chest x-ray
DIP — distal interphalangeal joint
DOE — dyspnea on exertion
EAH — exercise-associated hyponatremia
EBV — Epstein-Barr virus
EIA — exercise-induced asthma
EIB — exercise-induced bronchospasm
ECG — electrocardiogram
EMG — electromyelogram
EPB — extensor pollicis brevis
FABER — flexion, abduction, external rotation
FAT — female athlete triad
FDP — flexor digitorum profundus
FDS — flexor digitorum superficialis
fMRI — functional MRI
FOOSH — fall on outstretched hand
GERD — gastroesophageal reflux disease
GI — gastroentestinal
HR — heart rate
HCM — hypertrophic cardiomyopathy
HIV — human immunodeficiency virus
HPV — human papilloma virus
IOC — International Olympic Committee
IV — intravenous

IM — infectious mononucleosis
ITB — iliotibial band
LAC — long arm cast
LBM — lean body mass
LCL — lateral collateral ligament
LOC — loss of consciousness
MC — metacarpal
MCL — medial collateral ligament
MCP — metacarpophalangeal joint
MDI — multi-directional instability
MRI — magnetic resonance imaging
MRSA — methacillin-resistant *Staphlococcus aureus*
MTBI — mild traumatic brain injury
MTP — metatarsalphalangeal joint
MTSS — medial tibial stress syndrome
MV — mitral valve
NCAA — National Collegiate Athletic Association
NCS — nerve conduction study
NCV — nerve conduction velocity
NP — neuropsychiatric
NS — normal saline
NSAIDs — nonsteroidal anti-inflammatory drugs
OCD — osteochondritis dessicans
ORIF — open reduction, internal fixation
OTS — overtraining syndrome
PCL — posterior cruciate ligament
PCP — primary care provider
PCSS — post-concussion signs and symptoms
PFT — pulmonary function test
PIP — proximal interphalangeal joint
PPE — pre-participation exam
PPI — protein pump inhibitor
PRICE — protect, rest, ice, elevation
PT — physical therapy
PTA — post-traumatic amnesia
RC — rotator cuff
RGA — retrograde amnesia
RICE — rest, ice, compression, elevation
ROM — range of motion
RTP — return to play
SAC — short arm cast
SCD — sudden cardiac death

SCFE — slipped capital femoral epiphysis
SCM — sterno-cleido-mastoideus neck flexors
SD — standard deviation
SI — sacroiliac joint
SLAP — superior labrum anterior–posterior
SLC — short leg cast
TFCC — triangular fibrocartilaginous complex

TOS — thoracic outlet syndrome
US — ultrasound
USADA— U.S. Anti-doping Agency
USATF — U.S. Track and Field
VCD — vocal cord dysfunction
VL — vastus lateralis muscle
VMO — vastus medialis oblique muscle
WADA — World Anti-doping Association

I ■ INTRODUCTION

"Sports medicine" is a term that means different things to different people. For the context of this book, sports medicine will be defined as "medical care for the active individual." Though that definition is broad in its context, the field of sports medicine has its own uniqueness and holds a pertinent place in modern day health care delivery.

Sports medicine encompasses a variety of disciplines. The audience for this book is the non-surgeon practicing sports medicine, including primary care physicians, athletic trainers, and physical therapists.

Sports medicine is more than just management of musculoskeletal injuries; it is primary care medicine for the active individual, from the preschooler to the elderly tri-athlete. Primary care sports medicine includes not only the specialties of family medicine, pediatrics, internal medicine, physical medicine, and rehabilitation and emergency medicine, but also cardiology, pulmonology, nutrition, psychology, pharmacology, neurology, and others. Each of these specialties plays a role in the health of the active individual.

With the introduction of Primary Care Sports Medicine Fellowship programs in the late 1980s and early 1990s, primary care physicians were afforded sports medicine specialty training allowing them to take advantage of the different components of various medical disciplines that specifically apply to active individuals. The advent of a specialty exam (Certificate of Added Qualifications in Sports Medicine) allowed board certified primary specialists (Family Practice, Internal Medicine, Pediatrics, Emergency Medicine, and Physical Medicine and Rehabilitation) who completed an accredited fellowship in Sports Medicine to legitimately call themselves "sports medicine specialists." This relatively new field is advancing health care delivery to active individuals and is the focus of this book.

The core members of the sports medicine team, that provide the most frequent medical care for high school, college, professional, and Olympic athletes, include the certified athletic trainer, the primary care team physician, and the orthopedic consultant.

All three of these specialists are vital to the health of the athletes, but each may be the primary provider of medical care at different points in the delivery of health care (Fig. 1). The *athletic trainer* is often the person who sees to the daily maintenance of health care including advice on nutrition, first aid, and determination of need for consultation with the primary care team physician or orthopedic consultant. The *primary care team physician* performs pre-participation physical examinations, reviews past medical problems, and is responsible for the general medical care of the athletes and the treatment of musculoskeletal injuries. Depending on their level of experience, much of the required health care is performed by the team physician. If consultation is needed outside of the physician's training or comfort level, the team physician refers the athlete to the appropriate consultant. For musculoskeletal injuries, the team physician evaluates and treats the non-surgical conditions and refers potential surgical conditions to an *orthopedic consultant.*

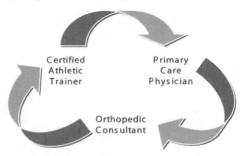

Certified Athletic Trainer

Primary Care Physician

Orthopedic Consultant

It must be emphasized that the training room is not a place for egotistical personalities. For a health care delivery system to work well, mutual respect and appreciation among the practitioners are vital to ensure that the health of the athlete remains the primary goal.

Another approach for viewing the care of the athlete is the "umbrella concept." In this analogy, the athlete is the stem of the umbrella while the individual ribs of the umbrella represent those on the sports medicine team who work together to make the athlete successful. These individuals include the above three specialists (certified athletic trainer, primary care team physician, and orthopedic consultant) as well as coaches, strength and conditioning professionals, physical therapists, nutritionists, sports psychologists, education counselors, and administrators.

II ■ PRE-PARTICIPATION EXAM

INTRODUCTION

The pre-participation exam (PPE) is a screening exam performed prior to sports participation. Although the style and selected portions of the exam differ among physicians, it still serves as a vital component of an athlete's health care.

The primary objective of the PPE is to screen athletes for any condition that may limit participation or that may place the athlete at risk for injury. It also screens for potentially life-threatening or disabling conditions and may be necessary to meet legal and insurance requirements. Secondary objectives include determining overall health, counseling athletes regarding health-related issues, and assessing fitness levels for specific sports. It should be remembered that, in many cases, this is the only exposure adolescents may have to health care.

Many states require a full screening exam on an annual basis. Ideal timing would be to perform the exam 4 to 6 weeks before sports participation in order to resolve or address any possible issues prior to beginning the activity. As a screening exam, it does not replace a comprehensive physical exam.

The following is an example of pertinent history questions and physical exam techniques.

HISTORY

Have the patient explain in detail any "yes" answers to the following questions.

1) Has a doctor ever denied or restricted your participation in sports for any reason?
2) Do you have an ongoing medical condition (like diabetes or asthma)?
3) Are you currently taking any prescription or non-prescription (over-the-counter) medications or supplements?
4) Do you have allergies to medications, pollens, foods, or stinging insects?
5) Have you ever passed out or nearly passed out *during* exercise?
6) Have you ever passed out or nearly passed out *after* exercise?
7) Have you ever had discomfort, pain, or pressure in your chest during exercise?
8) Does your heart race or skip beats during exercise?
9) Has doctor ever told you that you have (check all that apply):
   a) High BP
   b) Heart murmur
   c) High cholesterol
   d) Heart infection

10) Has a doctor ever ordered a test for your heart (i.e., ECG, echocardiogram)?
11) Has anyone in your family died for no apparent reason?
12) Does anyone in your family have a heart problem?
13) Has any family member or relative died suddenly or of heart problems before age 50?
14) Does anyone in your family have Marfan syndrome?
15) Have you ever spent the night in a hospital?
16) Have you ever had surgery?
17) Have you ever had an injury, such as a sprain, muscle or ligament tear, or tendonitis, that caused you to miss a practice or game?
18) Have you had any broken or fractured bones or dislocated joints?
19) Have you had a bone or joint injury that required x-rays, MRI, CT, surgery, injections, rehabilitation, physical therapy, or a brace, cast, or crutches?
20) Have you ever had a stress fracture?
21) Have you had an x-ray for, or been told that you have, atlantoaxial (neck) instability?
22) Do you regularly use a brace or assistive device?
23) Has a doctor ever told you that you have asthma or allergies?
24) Do you cough, wheeze, or have difficulty breathing during or after exercise?
25) Is there anyone in your family who has asthma?
26) Have you ever used an inhaler or taken asthma medicine?
27) Were you born without, or are you missing, a kidney, eye, testicle, or any other organ?
28) Have you had IM (mono) within the last month?
29) Do you have any rashes, pressure sores or other skin problems?
30) Have you had a herpes skin infection?
31) Have you ever had a head injury or concussion?
32) Have you been hit in the head and been confused or lost your memory?
33) Have you ever had a seizure?
34) Do you have headaches with exercise?
35) Have you ever had numbness, tingling, or weakness in your arms or legs after being hit or after falling?
36) Have you ever been unable to move your arms or legs after being hit or after falling?
37) When exercising in hot weather, do you have severe muscle cramps or become ill?
38) Has a doctor told you that you or someone in your family has sickle cell trait or sickle cell disease?
39) Have you had any problems with your eyes or vision?
40) Do you wear glasses or contact lenses?
41) Do you wear protective eyewear, such as goggles or a face shield?
42) Are you happy with your weight?

43) Are you trying to gain or lose weight?
44) Has anyone recommended you change your weight or eating habits?
45) Do you limit or carefully control what you eat?
46) Do you have any concerns that you would like to discuss with a doctor?

Females only:

47) Have you ever had a menstrual period?
48) How old were you when you had your first menstrual period?
49) How many periods have you had in the last 12 months?

PHYSICAL EXAM

This is only a screening exam; pertinent findings are to be examined in more depth.

- **Vitals:** Height, weight, BP, pulse
- **HEENT:** Visual acuity, pupil size
- **Neck:** Nodes
- **Lungs:** Wheeze, prolonged expiration, cough with forced expiration
- **CV:** Rate, rhythm, murmur, extra heart sounds (S3, S4)
  - *Murmurs:* Hypertrophic cardiomyopathy; intensity increased with standing or Valsalva; intensity decreased when squatting
  - *Aortic stenosis/innocent murmurs:* Intensity decreased with Valsalva; increased when squatting
- **Abdomen:** Masses, organomegaly
- **Skin:** Rashes, moles, lesions
- **Genitalia** (males only): Hernia, single/undescended testicle, testicular mass
- **Musculoskeletal:**
  - *Inspection:* With athlete standing, facing examiner: Check symmetry of trunk and upper extremities
  - *Neck:* Forward flexion, extension, rotation, and lateral flexion: Check ROM and cervical spine
  - *Shoulder:*
    a) Resisted shoulder shrug: Check trapezius strength
    b) Resisted shoulder abduction: Check deltoid strength
    c) Internal/external rotation of shoulder: Check ROM in glenohumeral joint
  - *Elbow:*
    a) Extension/flexion of elbow: Check ROM at elbow
    b) Pronation/supination of elbow: Check ROM at elbow and wrist
  - *Hand:* Clench fist then spread fingers: Check ROM in hand and fingers

- *Back/spine*:
    a) Back extension with knees straight: May be painful with spondylolysis/
       spondylolisthesis
    b) Back flexion with knees straight, facing toward and away from exam-
       iner: Check ROM in thoracic and lumbosacral spine, spine curvature
       and hamstring flexibility
- *Legs*:
    a) Inspection of lower extremities, contraction of quadriceps muscles:
       Check alignment and symmetry
    b) Athlete "duck walks" four steps: Check motion of hip, knee, and ankle,
       and strength and balance.
    c) Athlete stands on toes, then on heels: Check symmetry in calves and
       strength and balance

CARDIAC PHYSICAL EXAM

Answers to these cardiac screening questions will guide the practitioner
regarding the required extent of the cardiac physical examination. Particular
attention should be given to athletes who answer affirmatively regarding:
   1) Heart murmur
   2) High BP
   3) Chest pain/discomfort upon exertion
   4) Unexplained fainting or near-fainting
   5) Excessive and unexplained fatigue associated with exercise
Despite the low incidence of cardiovascular disease in an apparently healthy
athlete, a cardiac examination is vital to a pre-participation physical exam.
The American Heart Association recommends a screening cardiac exam be performed every 2 years, which requires careful tracking.

For the exam, the athlete should dress to allow ease in listening to the heart
and feeling the radial and femoral pulses. Boys should dress in shorts and girls
in shorts and sports bra or tank top. It is also crucial that the setting be quiet
enough to hear with auscultation.

The cardiac physical examination starts with obtaining a radial pulse and
resting BP, using an appropriately sized cuff, in the sitting position. Precordial
auscultation should be performed in the standing position and while supine
with and without a Valsalva maneuver. This assists in identifying heart murmurs consistent with dynamic left ventricular outflow obstruction. The femoral
artery pulses should be palpated to exclude coarctation of the aorta. Finally,
physical stigmata of Marfan syndrome should also be noted.

Auscultation should concentrate on the following five points:
   1) Listen to the *first heart sound* for intensity and apparent splitting. The
      first heart sound correlates with the length of the P-R interval on the
      ECG. Listening along the left sternal border determines normal split-
      ting. In the normal heart, left-sided events occur before those on the
      right side; hence, MV closure precedes tricuspid closure and accounts
      for the splitting of S 1.

2) Listen to the *second heart sound* for intensity and splitting. S2 corresponds to the closure of the aortic valve followed by the pulmonic valve. Listening at the left second or third interspace aids the practitioner. The sound normally is single in expiration and splits in inspiration.

3) Listen for *extra sounds in systole* such as the systolic click of MV prolapse or ejection sounds. Listen for *extra sounds in diastole* such as S3 or S4 or opening snaps. Record their location, pitch, intensity, timing and relationship to respiration.

4) Listen for *systolic murmurs*. Systolic murmurs occur between S1 and S2. Innocent or "functional" murmurs are a frequent finding in athletes and children during development. Characteristics of innocent murmurs include:

   a) the murmur is short, occurring early in systole and is not holosystolic

   b) the murmur is faint (grades 1 to 3).

5) Innocent murmurs are best heard in the supine position and should decrease with standing and Valsalva.

Listen for *diastolic murmurs*. Diastolic murmurs occur between S2 and S1. They are significant and indicate heart disease (i.e., mitral stenosis or aortic regurgitation).

CLUES TO HEART MURMURS:

1) If the first heart sound can be easily heard, the murmur is not holosystolic. Holosystolic murmurs are heard in ventricular septal defect and mitral insufficiency.

2) If a normal S2 is present, tetralogy of Fallot, atrial septal defect and pulmonary hypertension can be excluded. Listen for a normally split S2. An abnormally split S2 can be seen in tetralogy of Fallot, atrial septal defect and pulmonary hypertension.

3) If no ejection click exists, aortic and pulmonic stenoses are not present.

4) If there is no continuous diastolic murmur, patent ductus arteriosus is excluded.

5) If no early diastolic decrescendo murmur exists, aortic insufficiency is not present.

6) If normal femoral pulses are present, coarctation of the aorta does not exist.

SPECIAL TESTS IN MUSCULOSKELETAL MEDICINE

NECK

■ Spurling Maneuver (Foraminal Compression Test)

- **Purpose:** To determine if there is any foraminal compression caused by disc pathology or facet hypertrophy/arthritis causing neck or shoulder pain.

- **Description:** Apply mild cervical extension with lateral side bending, then rotate neck to one side and then the other while applying axial compression. Be sure to rule out a fracture prior to this test.
- **Positive Result:** Pain parasthesias or numbness radiating down the ipsilateral arm.

THORAX

■ Adson Maneuver
- **Purpose:** To evaluate for possible thoracic outlet syndrome.
- **Description:** Patient's arm is abducted and externally rotated while head is rotated toward the affected side.
- **Positive Result:** Reproduction of pain or sensory symptoms in the arm. Diminution or total loss of radial pulse is not uncommon and should not be considered a positive test.

■ Roos Maneuver
- **Purpose:** To check for possible thoracic outlet syndrome. Considered more accurate than the Adson maneuver.
- **Description:** Abduct arm to 90° and flex elbow to 90°. Have patient open and close hands repeatedly.
- **Positive Result:** Shoulder regional pain symptoms with the repeated motion.

SHOULDER

■ Apprehension Test
- **Purpose:** To test for stability of the glenohumeral joint.
- **Description:** Patient is in the supine position. Affected arm is abducted to 90°. With the elbow flexed at 90°, apply force to the forearm to externally rotate the arm and apply an anterior force to the humerus.
- **Positive Result:** Patient resists rotation or senses instability.

■ Crank Test
- **Purpose:** To examine for possible labral tear of the shoulder.
- **Description:** Elevate arm to approximately 160° and then provide forceful internal and external rotation.
- **Positive Result:** Pain and or clicking.

■ Cross-Body Adduction
- **Purpose:** To determine acromio-clavicular joint etiology.
- **Description:** Elevate the shoulder to 90° and adduct arm across the body.
- **Positive Result:** Indicates acromio-clavicular joint involvement.

■ Empty-Can Test
- **Purpose:** To assess supraspinatus tendonitis or partial or full-thickness tear.
- **Description:** Arm is abducted to 90° with forward flexion to 30° with thumb down. Apply downward stress to arm in that position.
- **Positive Result:** Pain and weakness to resistance.

■ **Hawkin Test**
- **Purpose:** To determine impingement of the subacromial space that includes the bursa and the supraspinatus tendon.
- **Description:** Flex the elbow to 90° and forward flex arm to 90°, then fully internally rotate the humerus so the hand is in front of the contralateral shoulder. With the arm in this position apply overpressure in internal rotation.
- **Positive Result:** Pain during the maneuver.

■ **Jobe Relocation Test**
- **Purpose:** To evaluate for shoulder instability.
- **Description:** Performed with patient in supine position and arm in 90° of abduction and external rotation. Examiner pushes anteriorly on the posterior aspect of the humeral head.
- **Positive Result:** Instability; a normal shoulder would be asymptomatic.

■ **Neer Test**
- **Purpose:** To determine impingement of the subacromial space.
- **Description:** Depress scapula with one hand and elevate arm to full forward flexion.
- **Positive Result:** Pain during the maneuver.

■ **O'Brien Test (Active Compression Test)**
- **Purpose:** To check for possible labral tear of the shoulder, particularly in the superior region.
- **Description:** Place the affected arm in 90° of forward flexion and 20° of cross-adduction. Have patient forward flex arm against resistance both with the thumb pointed upward and downward.
- **Positive Result:** If the discomfort is greater with the thumb downward, it is suggestive of a labral tear.

■ **Speed Test (Straight Arm Test)**
- **Purpose:** To check for biceps tendon injury.
- **Description:** Have patient move arm into forward flexion against resistance with the elbow straight and the palm upward.
- **Positive Result:** Pain, which indicates biceps tendon inflammation or injury.

■ **Sulcus Sign**
- **Purpose:** To determine if patient has inferior shoulder laxity.
- **Description:** Apply inferior traction to the affected arm.
- **Positive Result:** A sulcus will develop just below the acromion.

■ **Resisted Supination External Rotation Test**
- **Purpose:** To assess for possible labral tear
- **Description:** Patient is supine with scapula almost off edge of table. Arm is abducted to 90° and elbow is flexed to 50° to 60°. Have patient resist supination while externally rotating shoulder.
- **Positive Result:** Deep shoulder pain or clicking or catching in shoulder.

■ **Yergason Test**
- **Purpose:** To determine stability of biceps tendon in the bicipital groove.
- **Description:** Flex at elbow to 90°. Have patient leave arm at side and place hand on elbow and wrist. Have patient flex elbow and supinate the forearm against resistance.
- **Positive Result:** Biceps tendon slips out of bicipital groove or pain with examination.

ELBOW

■ **Lateral Epicondylitis Test**
- **Purpose:** To assess for possible lateral epicondylitis.
- **Description:** Have patient extend middle finger or wrist against resistance.
- **Positive Result:** Pain over the lateral epicondyle or common extensor tendon.

■ **Medial Epicondylitis Test**
- **Purpose:** To assess for possible medial epicondylitis.
- **Description:** Have patient flex wrist against resistance.
- **Positive Result:** Pain over the medial epicondyle or common flexor tendon.

■ **Milking Maneuver**
- **Purpose:** To assess the ulnar collateral ligament.
- **Description:** Abduct arm to 90° and flex elbow to 90°. Grab thumb and apply force medially.
- **Positive Result:** Pain with maneuver.

■ **Tinel Sign**
- **Purpose:** To assess ulnar nerve compression as it passes through the cubital tunnel that lies in the groove between the olecranon and the medial epicondyle.
- **Description:** Light tapping over the nerve.
- **Positive Result:** Pain and/or paresthesias over the ulnar border of the hand.

■ **Valgus Stress Test**
- **Purpose:** To assess the ulnar collateral ligament.
- **Description:** With arm at side, flex elbow roughly 30°. Place one hand on wrist and another over the elbow and apply valgus stress.
- **Positive Result:** Pain with maneuver or increased laxity compared to the other side.

WRIST AND HAND

■ **Finkelstein Test**
- **Purpose:** To assess for de Quervain tenosynovitis.
- **Description:** Have patient make a fist with thumb inserted inside the fingers. Place patient in ulnar deviation.
- **Positive Result:** Pain at radial aspect of wrist at time of exam.

- ■ **Grind Test**
  - **Purpose:** To assess for possible thumb carpometacarpal joint arthritis.
  - **Description:** Place patient hand in relaxed supination. Grasp the MC base and rotate the thumb carpo MC joint while applying axial compression.
  - **Positive Result:** Pain with this motion.
- ■ **Phalen Maneuver**
  - **Purpose:** To assess for possible carpal tunnel syndrome.
  - **Description:** Have patient place hands in gravity flexion of wrists.
  - **Positive Result:** Pain or paresthesia in distribution of median nerve.
- ■ **Radial and Ulnar Collateral Ligament Tests**
  - **Purpose:** To assess the radial and ulnar collateral ligaments along each finger or thumb.
  - **Description:** Take the injured finger or thumb and apply varus and valgus over the proximal interphalangeal joint at 30° flexion.
  - **Positive Result:** Pain or laxity with maneuver.
- ■ **Tinel Sign**
  - **Purpose:** To assess for possible carpal tunnel syndrome.
  - **Description:** Lightly tap the median nerve at the wrist flexion crease at same plane as 2nd MC.
  - **Positive Result:** Pain or paresthesia in distribution of median nerve.

LUMBAR SPINE

- ■ **Crossed Straight Leg Raise Test**
  - **Purpose:** To assess for a possible nerve root impingement caused by a herniated disc. Tests for neural tension and radiculopathy.
  - **Description:** With patient supine, raise unaffected leg above 60° to 70°.
  - **Positive Result:** Pain in the affected leg that recreates radicular symptoms.
- ■ **One Leg Standing Hyperextension Test (Stork Test)**
  - **Purpose:** To assess for possible spondylolysis, spondylolisthesis, or sacroiliac dysfunction.
  - **Description:** Have patient stand and lift leg on side of pain. At same time have patient hyperextend back.
  - **Positive Result:** Pain in the lumbar spine.
- ■ **Seated Straight Leg Raise Test**
  - **Purpose:** To assess for a possible nerve root impingement. This test is used as secondary tool because patients with a positive supine straight leg raise should also have pain with a seated straight leg raise. A positive straight leg raise and a negative seated straight leg raise should raise suspicion.
  - **Description:** With patient seated, have neck placed in flexion and lift leg in same manner as straight leg raise (see below).
  - **Positive Result:** Pain when affected leg is raised 60° to 70° and recreates radicular symptoms.

- **Straight Leg Raise Test**
  - **Purpose:** To assess for a possible nerve root impingement caused by a herniated disc.
  - **Description:** With patient supine, the examiner raises affected leg.
  - **Positive Result:** Pain when affected leg is raised above 60° to 70° and recreates radicular symptoms.

HIP

- **FABER Test (Patrick Test)**
  - **Purpose:** To detect possible sacroiliac joint pathology.
  - **Description:** Place the supine patient in position by FABER (**F**lexing, **AB**ducting and **E**xternally **R**otating the hip). Because this is done with the knee flexed, it is also called the "figure four" exam.
  - **Positive Result:** Pain with this motion.

- **Hip Flexion Test**
  - **Purpose:** To assess for possible slipped capital femoral epiphysis or joint incongruity.
  - **Description:** In supine position, observe hip rotation while patient flexes hips.
  - **Positive Result:** Compulsory external rotation.

- **Log Roll Test**
  - **Purpose:** To determine if there is any pathology affecting the hip joint including infection, fracture, or synovitis.
  - **Description:** In supine position, with legs in full extension, gently roll the legs to internal and external rotation.
  - **Positive Result:** Exquisite pain with rolling motion.

KNEE

- **Anterior Drawer Test**
  - **Purpose:** To assess for a torn ACL.
  - **Description:** Patient is supine with knees bent to 90° and feet placed flat on the examination table. Stabilize foot and gently pull the proximal lower leg forward.
  - **Positive Result:** Anterior translation of tibia on femur with no definitive endpoint.

- **Apley Compression Test**
  - **Purpose:** To assess for a possible meniscal tear.
  - **Description:** Place patient in prone position. Knee is flexed to 90° and internal and external rotation is applied by twisting the ankle and applying axial compression force through the bottom of the heel.
  - **Positive Result:** Pain with compression.

■ **Lachman Test**
  • **Purpose:** To assess for a torn ACL.
  • **Description:** With patient supine, hold the leg above the knee with your outside hand and just below the knee with your inside hand. Flex the knee to 20° or 30° and gently attempt to translate the tibia on the femur.
  • **Positive Result:** Increased anterior translation of the tibia on the femur without a solid endpoint. This is considered the "gold standard" in assessment for an ACL tear.

■ **McMurray Test**
  • **Purpose:** To check for a possible meniscal tear.
  • **Description:** With patient supine, place thumb and third finger over both medial and lateral joint lines. Hold the ankle with the other hand using it to flex and extend the knee while applying internal and external rotation.
  • **Positive Result:** Pain with this motion is considered positive but a more specific sign is pain with a palpable click at the joint line.

■ **Noble Compression Test**
  • **Purpose:** To assess for ITB syndrome.
  • **Description:** Place patient in supine position. Take affected leg in flexed position and place thumb with pressure proximal to lateral condyle and move into extension.
  • **Positive Result:** Pain between 30° and 40° extension.

■ **Ober Test**
  • **Purpose:** To assess ITB tightness.
  • **Description:** Place patient on unaffected side. Flex hip and then flex knee to 90°. Allow the patient to drop the knee as low as possible.
  • **Positive Result:** Patient cannot drop flexed knee below horizontal.

■ **Patellar Grind Test**
  • **Purpose:** To assess for chondromalacia associated with patellofemoral syndrome.
  • **Description:** Patient is in supine position and knee is fully extended. Examiner places hand over superior pole of kneecap and patient then tightens the quadriceps muscle.
  • **Positive Result:** Pain with maneuver or an associated crepitus.

■ **Pivot Shift Test**
  • **Purpose:** To assess for a torn ACL.
  • **Description:** Patient is supine. Knee is fully extended. Examiner places valgus stress along with internal rotation to knee while flexing knee joint.
  • **Positive Result:** Tibial subluxation or a "jump" near 90° of knee flexion.

■ **Posterior Drawer Test**
  • **Purpose:** To assess for a torn posterior cruciate ligament.
  • **Description:** Patient is supine and knee is flexed to 90°. Place hands over the proximal tibia with foot secured on examining table and apply pressure.
  • **Positive Result:** No endpoint and increased posterior laxity.

■ **Posterior Sag Sign**
- **Purpose:** To assess for a torn posterior cruciate ligament.
- **Description:** Patient is supine and knee is flexed to 90°.
- **Positive Result:** Posterior translation of tibia on femur.

■ **Steinman Test**
- **Purpose:** To assess for a possible meniscal tear.
- **Description:** Place patient in seated position on examination table. Grab ankle and perform internal and external rotation.
- **Positive Result:** Pain with internal and external rotation.

■ **Thessaly Test**
- **Purpose:** To assess for a possible meniscal tear.
- **Description:** Have patient stand. Provide some support while patient bends knees to 20° of flexion and provides rotational force at knee.
- **Positive Result:** Pain with internal and external rotation.

■ **Varus/Valgus Test**
- **Purpose:** To assess for a sprains of LCL/MCL.
- **Description:** Patient is supine. Examiner places valgus and varus stress across knee joint at 0° and 30° flexion.
- **Positive Result:** Pain and/or increased laxity.

ANKLE

■ **Anterior Drawer Test**
- **Purpose:** To determine increased joint laxity of the anterior talofibular ligament.
- **Description:** Grasp the patient at distal tibia to stabilize the lower extremity. With the other hand, grasp the heel with index finger on heel and thumb on anterior ankle mortise, and apply anterior force.
- **Positive Result:** Increased anterior laxity compared with the other ankle.

■ **External Rotation Stress Test**
- **Purpose:** To assess for a possible syndesmotic or injury to anterior tibio-fibular ligament (high ankle sprain).
- **Description:** Patient is seated with leg over table and knee flexed to 90°. Stabilize tibia with one hand and externally rotate foot.
- **Positive Result:** Pain with maneuver at anterior tibiofibular ligament or syndesmoses.

■ **Peroneal Stress Test**
- **Purpose:** To assess for peroneal tendon subluxation.
- **Description:** Patient is seated with leg over table and knee flexed to 90°. Have patient dorsiflex and evert ankle against resistance.
- **Positive Result:** Peroneal tendon subluxation or dislocation.

■ **Squeeze Test**
- **Purpose:** To check for a possible syndesmotic or high ankle sprain.
- **Description:** Place hands on patient's mid-calf and squeeze the tibia and fibula together.
- **Positive Result:** Pain that radiates down tibiofibular joint in lower leg.

■ **Talar Tilt Test**
- **Purpose:** To assess for injury to calcaneofibular ligament.
- **Description:** Position one hand over distal tibia and the other over the arch of midfoot. Apply inversion stress to heel and ankle.
- **Positive Result:** Increased laxity with soft or no endpoint.

■ **Thompson Squeeze Test**
- **Purpose:** To determine if there is a full-thickness tear of the Achilles tendon.
- **Description:** Place hands at mid-calf with patient prone. Squeeze the calf muscle and assess for passive plantar flexion of the ankle.
- **Positive Result:** No plantar flexion of the ankle, indicating a full-thickness tear of the tendon.

III ■ MUSCULOSKELETAL COMMON INJURIES

CERVICAL

■ Burners/Stingers
- **Definition:** Nerve injury or compression resulting from trauma to the neck or shoulder area. Can be caused by traction or compression along the brachial plexus or cervical nerve roots.
- **Mechanism of Injury:** Traction occurs when the shoulder is depressed while the neck is laterally flexed to the opposite side. Compression occurs with forceful lateral flexion and extension of the cervical spine.
- **Clinical Symptoms:** Immediate onset of burning pain down the arm unilaterally. It is associated with numbness or weakness.
- **Radiographs:** Cervical spine series, including flexion and extension views may be helpful, but are usually normal.
- **Treatment:** Symptomatic for pain and close follow up. Consider other diagnoses with bilateral or lower extremity involvement.

■ Cervical Strain/Sprain
- **Definition:** Partial or complete tear of the muscle (strain) or ligaments (sprain) around the neck.
- **Mechanism of Injury:** Cervical flexion, extension, rotation, side bending, or combination motion.
- **Clinical Symptoms:** Pain with active or passive motion, decreased ROM, paraspinal muscle spasms or tenderness. No numbness or tingling.
- **Radiographs:** Cervical spine series is indicated to rule out fracture if there is bony tenderness. In sprain/strain, the most common finding is loss of cervical lordosis due to muscle spasm.
- **Treatment:** Rest, ice, NSAIDs, physical therapy modalities, and muscle relaxants. Limit contact sports if decreased ROM or significant pain.

■ Cervical Spinal Stenosis
- **Definition:** Decreased sagittal diameter of the cervical spinal canal that may predispose an athlete to spinal cord injury in athletic trauma.
- **Mechanism of Injury:** Congenital or acquired (i.e., osteoarthritis).
- **Clinical Symptoms:** Often asymptomatic until injury occurs. With hyperflexion, hyperextension or axial load, the spinal cord may be compressed secondary to decreased diameter. C5 or C6 is most common. May result in unilateral neuropraxia, transient bilateral parasthesia with or without muscle weakness, or quadriparesis with arm weakness greater than leg weakness due to bruising of central spinal cord (central cord syndrome).
- **Radiographs:** Plain films suggest narrowing of the cervical spine. The Torg ratio measures the spinal canal diameter to vertebral body diameter.

A ratio of <0.8 suggests spinal stenosis, but is not universally accepted for competitive athletes. An MRI scan is more accurate for assessment.
- **Treatment:** Treatment ranges from observation, use of functional cervical collar, corticosteroid injection or surgical decompression.

THORACIC

- **Costochondritis**
  - **Definition:** Inflammation of the costocartilage that attaches from the end of the bony rib to the sternum.
  - **Mechanism of Injury:** May be due to direct trauma but often seen in the absence of trauma. Etiology often unclear; some suspect it is secondary to antecedent viral infection. May have costovertebral dysfunction.
  - **Clinical Symptoms:** Pain with direct palpation of the area or over the costal cartilage adjacent to the sternum. Often point specific. Pain increases with deep breath.
  - **Radiographs:** Radiographs not indicated unless there is suspicion of rib fracture.
  - **Treatment:** Ice or heat, rest, NSAIDs.

- **Idiopathic Scoliosis**
  - **Definition:** Lateral curvature of the spine >10°.
  - **Mechanism of Injury:** Etiology unknown. Often hereditary.
  - **Clinical Symptoms:** Often no symptoms and unrecognized for years. Frequently presents in adolescence and, once recognized, should be followed. Evaluated by back asymmetry and presence of rib hump with forward flexion (Adam test).
  - **Radiographs:** PA and lateral views of the thoracic spine. Axial skeletal maturity can be evaluated by looking for iliac crest apophysis ossification (Risser sign). Progression of curvature is less likely after skeletal maturity. Should be referred to a scoliosis expert.
  - **Treatment:** If <20°, follow with serial x-rays every 3 to 6 months. If moderate (20° to 40°) or progressive, bracing can decrease progression. Severe curvature requires spinal fusion with instrumentation.

- **Scapulothoracic Dysfunction/Dyskinesis**
  - **Definition:** Abnormality of scapulothoracic motion. SICK scapula acronym stands for: **S**capula malposition, **I**nferior medial border prominence, **C**oracoid pain and malposition and dys**K**inesis of scapular movement.
  - **Mechanism of Injury:** Often occurs in throwers or swimmers who present with shoulder pain. Caused by fatigue or abnormal shoulder mechanics; may be related to abnormal firing of the serratus anterior or middle or lower trapezius. Often occurs due to strain of the RC, which develops compensatory changes.
  - **Clinical Symptoms:** At rest, the scapula demonstrates asymmetries with the affected shoulder depressed and the scapula protracted. Scapular winging occurs with prominence of medial border of scapula. Abnormal scapulothoracic motion is observed from behind when the patient fully flexes or abducts the shoulder joint overhead. Crepitation may be heard or

palpated and may be related to reactive bursa (scapulothoracic bursitis). Patients present with dull, deep, achy pain.
- **Radiographs:** Routine shoulder films or scapular films are normal and usually unnecessary.
- **Treatment:** Initial treatment with rest, ice, NSAIDs, and physical therapy. Correction of dyskinesis with stretching and eventual strengthening of the posterior shoulder girdle and scapular stabilizers.

■ Scheuermann Disease
- **Definition:** Thoracic kyphosis with or without back pain. Seems to present in early adolescence and occurs from pressure or trauma to the anterior vertebral endplates that are still maturing, resulting in anterior compression of the vertebral bodies.
- **Mechanism of Injury:** Unknown etiology.
- **Clinical Symptoms:** Thoracic kyphosis that cannot be corrected by adjusting the posture. Occurs most commonly around T7.
- **Radiographs:** Lateral spine view shows anterior wedging of thoracic vertebrae, Schmorl nodes, and vertebral endplate irregularity. Typical Scheuermann disease involves three successive vertebrae; atypical Scheuermann disease does not and pain is more severe.
- **Treatment:** Mild cases are often asymptomatic and require no treatment. More significant cases require early recognition and treatment with Milwaukee brace followed by supervised exercise program.

LUMBAR

■ Degenerative Disease of the Lumbar Spine
- **Definition:** Tearing of the outer fibers of the annulus fibrosis in the posterolateral portion of the disc and herniation of the nucleus pulposus. Occurs most commonly at the L5-S1 or L4-5 discs between 30 and 40 years of age.
- **Mechanism of Injury:** Repetitive flexion and rotation stress increases intradiscal pressure. Often aggravated by abnormal lifting techniques with forward bending of the spine without use of the legs.
- **Clinical Symptoms:** Low back pain with radicular symptoms along a dermatomal pattern due to nerve root compression. Pain worsened with prolonged sitting and forward spine flexion. Large central disc herniation may affect bowel, bladder, or sexual function (cauda equina syndrome). Decreased ROM, often with list to one side in attempt to decrease nerve root pressure. Positive straight leg test. May have lower extremity weakness, decreased deep tendon reflexes, or sensory changes in corresponding dermatome. Annular tear without disc extrusion may present with significant back pain and muscle spasm.
- **Radiographs:** PA, lateral, and oblique films are often normal or may show decreased disc space. MRI indicated and may reveal disc herniation or associated disc desiccation and narrowing of the disc space.
- **Treatment:** Initial treatment is relative rest, ice, and physical therapy modalities. Some clinicians prefer oral or IM injectable corticosteroids

instead of NSAIDs. Epidural steroid injections indicated for those who do not respond to conservative measures. Surgical consultation and dissectomy indicated for those who fail the above approach.

■ **Facet Syndrome**
- **Definition:** Irritation of the spinal facet due to degenerative changes or inflammation.
- **Mechanism of Injury:** Etiology unclear but often degenerative or traumatic.
- **Clinical Symptoms:** Pain in low back, hip, or buttock, often aggravated with extension.
- **Radiographs:** PA, lateral, and oblique films may show degenerative changes or foraminal narrowing. CT or MRI may be indicated.
- **Treatment:** Initial treatment is relative rest, ice, NSAIDs, and progressive exercise program. Facet joint steroid injection may be beneficial. Medial branch blocks followed by nerve ablation may be indicated.

■ **Mechanical Low Back Pain**
- **Definition:** Non-specific lumbar pain related to the sprain or strain of otherwise normal tissue. Should be differentiated from structural, degenerative, or inflammatory low back pain associated with demonstrable tissue pathology. This is a "waste basket" diagnosis (i.e., a diagnosis of exclusion) usually applied early in the evaluation of back pain. If the pain persists, it is more likely that a specific pathologic diagnosis will be made.
- **Mechanism of Injury:** Improper lifting techniques (straight legs with back flexed), bending, or traumatic cause.
- **Clinical Symptoms:** Low back pain with limited ROM, with or without muscle spasm and a normal neurologic exam.
- **Radiographs:** Usually not indicated unless back pain persists. If pain persists 4 to 6 weeks, obtain AP, lateral, and oblique views.
- **Treatment:** Acute treatment involves ice, NSAIDs, avoidance of aggravating activity, and physical therapy modalities. Avoid prolonged bed rest. Use of narcotics or muscle relaxants should be done sparingly. Hamstring flexibility, proper lifting techniques, core and progressive extension strengthening, and aerobic conditioning are essential to prevent recurrences. Manual therapy or spinal adjustments.

■ **Sacroiliac Dysfunction**
- **Definition:** Pain over the SI joint that may mimic mechanical low back pain or discogenic disease.
- **Mechanism of Injury:** May have traumatic etiology or present secondary to herniated disc of lumbar strain.
- **Clinical Symptoms:** Pain over the sacroiliac joint, usually unilateral and/or with knee-to-chest motion that places unilateral stress on the joint. Pain is aggravated with pressure over the SI joint or FABER (hip **f**lexion, **ab**duction and **e**xternal **r**otation) of the unilateral leg.
- **Radiographs:** AP pelvic films usually normal.

- **Treatment:** Ice, NSAIDs, physical therapy modalities, and manipulation. Corticosteroid injection are often helpful for diagnosis or treatment.

■ Spondylolisthesis

- **Definition:** Forward slippage of one vertebra on the vertebra below it. Most commonly occurs at L5-S1. Slippage measured by degree of superior vertebral body displacement on the inferior vertebral body.
  - *Grade I:* 0 to 25%
  - *Grade II:* 25% to 50%
  - *Grade III:* 50% to 75%
  - *Grade IV:* 75% to 100%
- **Mechanism of Injury:** Repetitive stress, usually hyperextension, weakens the pars interarticularis. Common in gymnasts, football linemen, and volleyball athletes.
- **Clinical Symptoms:** Low back pain, tight hamstring, pain with extension, limitation of forward flexion. Usually normal neurologic exam. Palpable step-off may be present.
- **Radiographs:** PA, lateral, and oblique views. Oblique views reveal bilateral spondylolysis. Lateral views will grade degree of slippage, although flexion/extension films are important to determine instability. AP film may show superior slipped vertebra overlying inferior vertebra ("Napoleon's hat"). Bone scan, SPECT scan, or thin sliced CT may aid in diagnosis.
- **Treatment:** Most grade I slippages are treated conservatively with same treatment as spondylolysis. Serial radiographs are needed to follow slippage. Consider surgical fusion if slippage progresses. Spinal stenosis, nerve root compression, and pseudoclaudication may be complications of progressive or high-grade slippage.

■ Spondylolysis

- **Definition:** Fatigue or "stress" fracture of the pars interarticularis (bony segment between the superior and inferior articulating processes).
- **Mechanism of Injury:** Repetitive stress, usually hyperextension, weakens the pars interarticularis. Common in gymnasts, football linemen, and volleyball athletes.
- **Clinical Symptoms:** Low back pain off the midline. Worse with hyperextension and relieved by rest. Pain reproduced with one-leg hyperextension (stork test) or aggravated with side bending and rotation. No sciatic symptoms. May have bilateral symptoms.
- **Radiographs:** AP, lateral, and oblique views. Oblique view reveals a "Scotty dog" sign and may show the spondylitic fracture. Bone scan may be indicated if plain radiographs are negative and clinical suspicion persists. Thin slice CT may give better visualization. MRI with fat suppression may be more specific.
- **Treatment:** Treatment is dependent on radiographic findings.
  - *Normal plain films with positive bone scan:* Acute injury. Limit activity, institute core strengthening, medication, and modalities for pain relief.

- *Positive plain film and positive bone scan*: Semi-acute injury. Consider thermoplastic brace, although bracing is controversial. May participate in some sports with a brace. Limit activity and institute core strengthening as pain permits. Must have pain-free ROM to return to sports.
- *Positive plain films and negative bone scan*: Chronic injury. Probably means healing has occurred with a fibrous union. Core strengthening and progress to RTP as pain permits.
- *Persistent cases*: Consider surgical fusion.

PROCEDURES

■ Trigger Points Injection
- **Indications:** Myofascial trigger pain/points.
- **Patient Position:** Dependent upon location of trigger point, often fusiform firm nodule running parallel to muscle fibers. Must know local anatomy.
- **Technique:** Identify area and trap with fingers of non-dominant hand. Insert needle perpendicularly into center of tender trigger point.
- **Medicine/Needle:** 0-0.5 mL steroid/1-5 mL anesthetic or sterile saline.

SHOULDER INJURIES

OVERVIEW

■ Pain
- *Acute (less than 2 weeks)*: Fracture, dislocation, RC tear, bicep rupture, subacromial bursitis, RC tendonitis.
- *Chronic*: AC arthritis, degenerative glenohumeral joint arthritis, frozen shoulder, cervical root irritation.

■ Instability
Determine if partial (subluxation) or complete (dislocation). Determine location: anterior (traumatic), posterior, inferior, or multidirectional.

■ ROM/Muscle Strength/Functional Tests:
Compare active and passive ROM. Compare strength to unaffected side.

■ Age of Patient
- *Younger (<30)*: Tendonitis, dislocations, instability.
- *Older (>50)*: Impingement, RC tears, adhesive capsulitis, degenerative arthritis.

■ Radiographs
AP, lateral, scapular Y, axillary.

COMMON SHOULDER INJURIES

■ **Acromioclavicular Sprains, "Shoulder Separation"**
  • **Definition:** Stretch or tear of AC or CC (Costoclavicular) ligaments.
  • **Classification:** Based on severity and degree of clavicular separation.
    ◦ *Type I:* Sprain of AC ligament, CC ligaments intact, AC joint intact.
    ◦ *Type II:* Tear of AC ligament, sprain of CC ligaments, mild to moderate AC separation.
    ◦ *Type III:* Tear of AC and CC ligaments, AC joint separation 25% to 100%.
    ◦ *Type IV:* Complete AC dislocation with distal clavicle displaced posteriorly into trapezius muscle.
    ◦ *Type V:* Exaggerated Type III with 100% to 300% displacement of AC joint.
    ◦ *Type VI:* Complete AC dislocation with distal clavicle displaced inferiorly.
  • **Mechanism of Injury:** Fall on point of shoulder or outstretched hand.
  • **Clinical Symptoms:** Pain on palpation and shoulder movement, deformity, swelling. Positive crossover test or cross arm adduction.
  • **Radiographs:** AP views with 10° to 15° of cephalic tilt. Stress or weighted views may help differentiate degree of displacement.
  • **Treatment:**
    ◦ *Types I and II:* Ice, rest, sling, analgesics, ROM and strengthening exercise as pain permits. Figure-of-8 brace, sling, NSAIDs.
    ◦ *Type III:* Controversy between conservative versus surgical management.
    ◦ *Types IV, V, and VI:* Surgical reconstruction.

■ **Adhesive Capsulitis, "Frozen Shoulder"**
  • **Definition:** Restriction of ROM of the shoulder caused by adhesions and contraction of the shoulder capsule.
  • **Mechanism of Injury:** Often idiopathic, but more frequent in diabetics. Etiology unclear, but often presents with voluntary then persistent restrictions in motion after minor shoulder trauma.
  • **Clinical Symptoms:** Pain and loss of active and passive range of shoulder motion. Often keeps the patient from sleeping. Usually occurs in older (>40 years) patients.
  • **Radiographs:** Routine radiographs are usually normal.
  • **Treatment:** NSAIDs with gentle ROM exercises and moist heat are used initially. An intra-articular or subacromial corticosteroid injection may be beneficial. For recalcitrant cases, surgical manipulation under anesthesia to break adhesions followed by prompt physical therapy are indicated.

■ **Biceps Tendonitis/Biceps Tendon Rupture**
  • **Definition:** The long head of the biceps tendon is subject to inflammation from associated RC impingement. Occasionally the tendon may sublux out of the bicipital groove.
  • **Mechanism of Injury:** Chronic overhead activity. Biceps tendonitis is associated with impingement syndrome. Occasionally the biceps tendon can rupture with forced elbow flexion revealing retraction of the muscle belly and a "Popeye" deformity.

- **Clinical Symptoms**: Pain with activity or nighttime pain. Positive forward flexion or horizontal abduction with Speed or Yergason tests.
- **Radiographs**: Routine radiographs are usually normal.
- **Treatment**: Rest, ice, NSAIDs with physical therapy. Repair of a biceps tendon rupture is not recommended in older patients. Surgical tenodesis may be indicated in younger patients.

■ **Brachial Plexopathy, "Burners/Stingers"**
- **Definition**: Neurologic injury involving transient motor and/or sensory loss of the upper extremity.
- **Mechanism of Injury**: Traction or compression injuries of the upper cervical nerve roots, usually C5-6. Injuries are common in American football but may also occur in other contact sports. Stretch injuries may occur with downward shoulder pressure, forcing the neck to the opposite side. Compression injuries may be secondary to stenosis as the nerve roots exit the cervical foramen. This carries a worse prognosis.
- **Clinical Symptoms**: Sharp pain with a burning sensation that extends down the arm with associated weakness. Often the individual will exit the field with the arm hanging at the side.
- **Radiographs**: Routine radiographs are usually normal. With recurrent compression injuries look for foraminal stenosis on oblique views. If symptoms persist, EMG and MRI may be indicated.
- **Treatment**: Single episodes that resolve with restoration of ROM, sensation, and strength permit return to normal activity. For repeated episodes or compression type, further studies should be considered to disclose cervical disc disease or foraminal stenosis.

■ **Clavicle Fractures**
- **Definition**: Most common location is the middle third of the clavicle.
- **Mechanism of Injury**: Fall on point of shoulder or outstretched hand.
- **Clinical Symptoms**: Visible/palpable deformity. Pain, swelling, ecchymosis to anterior chest. Spasm of upper trapezius or neck.
- **Radiographs**: AP and axillary views. Consider CXR to rule out pneumothorax. Evaluate for scapula fracture if indicted.
- **Treatment**: Sling, figure-of-8 brace, ice, analgesics, rest.

■ **Glenohumeral Arthritis**
- **Definition**: Loss of joint space caused by destruction of the glenohumeral articular cartilage.
- **Mechanism of Injury**: Post-traumatic arthritis, rheumatoid arthritis, osteoarthritis, arthropathy secondary to long-term RC tears.
- **Clinical Symptoms**: Limited ROM and pain that starts with normal activity and later progresses to pain at night and at rest. Crepitation with ROM.
- **Radiographs**: AP and axillary views reveal joint space narrowing, osteophytes, and subchondral erosions.
- **Treatment**: Initial treatment includes ice or heat, NSAIDs, and gentle ROM exercises. Cortisone injections prove to be of temporary benefit. Surgical options include total shoulder replacement or hemiarthroplasty.

■ **Glenohumeral Instability, "Shoulder Dislocation"**
- **Definition:** The shoulder sacrifices "stability" for "mobility." The shoulder can sublux (partial dislocation or partial separation of the articular surfaces) or dislocate (complete translation of the articular surfaces). Instability can occur in the following directions: anterior, posterior, inferior, or multidirectional. MDI and anterior are the most common. MDI uses the acronym "AMBRI" [atraumatic, multidirectional, bilateral, rehabilitation (used initially for treatment) and inferior capsular shift as the preferred surgical procedure]. Anterior instability uses the acronym "TUBS" (traumatic, unilateral, Bankart, surgery). A Bankart lesion is a tear of the anterior glenoid labrum.
- **Mechanism of Injury:** The usual method of dislocation includes extension, abduction, and external rotation.
- **Clinical Symptoms:** The patient describes a sensation of the shoulder slipping in the joint associated with pain and apprehension.
- **Radiographs:** AP, axillary, and scapular Y views. Axillary view may reveal a bony Bankart lesion (a chip fracture off of the anterior inferior glenoid). A Hill-Sachs lesion involves a compression fracture of the posterior humeral head. An MRI arthrogram may be indicated to reveal a labral tear.
- **Treatment:** Initial anterior dislocations require prompt reduction. It is appropriate to attempt an on-field reduction if the neurovascular status is normal and there is no clinical evidence of a fracture associated with the dislocation. The arm should be placed in a sling and post-reduction radiographs should be obtained. The arm should remain in the sling for comfort for 1 to 2 weeks. ROM exercises and RC strengthening should begin when pain resolves. Return to sport requires full ROM and near normal strength. Surgery is indicated for recurrent dislocators, though there is strong evidence to indicate better results may occur with early repair after the first dislocation.

■ **Glenoid Labral Tears**
- **Definition:** The labrum is the soft tissue cushion between the bony glenoid and the humeral head.
- **Mechanism of Injury:** A labral tear can be traumatic secondary to a dislocation or as a result of chronic overuse resulting in partial tears and fraying. During the acceleration phase of throwing or pitching, horizontal adduction and internal rotation can grind the labrum resulting in a SLAP lesion. (A "SLAP" lesion refers to a tear of the Superior Labrum from Anterior to Posterior.) In the cocked position, the RC is pinched against the posterior labrum resulting in fraying. Abnormal forces on the labrum can result from asynchronous firing of the RC or weakness of the posterior cuff muscles.
- **Clinical Symptoms:** Positional pain, sometimes with an abnormal click or clunk. Decrease in throwing velocity is often reported.
- **Radiographs:** Routine radiographs are usually normal unless a bony Bankart lesion is present. An MRI arthrogram will reveal the labral tear.

- **Treatment:** Initial treatment includes ice, rest, NSAIDs, and physical therapy. With failure of the above treatment, arthroscopic repair or debridement of the labrum is indicated followed by appropriate rehabilitation.

■ **Proximal Humeral Fractures**
- **Definition:** Proximal humerus fractures are delineated by the area of injury: 1) greater tuberosity, 2) lesser tuberosity, 3) humeral head, and 4) shaft. Further classification involves the anatomic or surgical neck.
- **Mechanism of Injury:** FOOSH or falling directly on the shoulder. More common in older people with osteoporotic bone. Less common in young people, but can occur with violent trauma.
- **Clinical Symptoms:** Pain, bruising, and swelling of the proximal arm. Patient holds arm splinted against body. Neurovascular status must be evaluated: numbness may indicate axillary nerve injury, whereas decreased pulse or paleness may indicate injury to the axillary artery.
- **Radiographs:** AP, scapular Y, and axillary views are necessary. CT is indicated if fracture is suspected, but hard to visualize on x-ray.
- **Treatment:** Minimally displaced (<1 cm) injuries can be treated conservatively with sling immobilization and early ROM. Injuries with displacement >1 cm should receive surgical consideration.

■ **Rotator Cuff Impingement (Tendonitis/Tendinosis/Subacromial Bursitis)**
- **Definition:** The RC consists of the following tendons: subscapularis, supraspinatus, infraspinatus and teres minor. Inflammation of these tendons, most commonly the supraspinatus, associated with swelling in the subacromial bursae impinges on the coracoacromial ligament and the undersurface of the acromion.
- **Mechanism of Injury:** Overuse of the shoulder associated with RC weakness and/or repetitive overhead activities. Primary impingement is caused by bony pathology from downsloping acromion or AC osteophytes. Secondary impingement occurs in a normal space that is decreased from ligamentous laxity and poor RC stabilization of the glenohumeral joint.
- **Clinical Symptoms:** Pain aggravated by overhead motion. Pain at night is especially prominent in bursitis.
- **Radiographs:** Routine radiographs may be normal or may show a subacromial spur or arthritis and spurring of the AC joint. Evidence of calcific tendonitis may be seen primarily in the supraspinatus tendon. A suprascapular outlet view can reveal the shape of the acromion to be Type I (flat), Type II (curved) or Type III (hooked).
- **Treatment:** Ice, NSAIDs, and restriction of overhead or aggravating motion is indicated initially. Physical therapy is used to restore ROM and strength. A subacromial injection with 10 cc of 1% lidocaine may confirm the diagnosis, whereas a subacromial cortisone injection may decrease the inflammation and initiate healing. Subacromial decompression via arthroscopy is indicated for persistent cases.

- ■ **Rotator Cuff Tears**
  - **Definition:** The RC, particularly the supraspinatus, may be involved in a partial or full thickness tear resulting in discontinuity of tendon fibers and is associated with weakness, inflammation, and pain.
  - **Mechanism of Injury:** Overuse leads to tendonitis and tendonisis. *Acute tears* may result from a direct blow or indirect force to the abducted arm. *Chronic tears* result from long term inflammation and gradual weakening of the tendon fibers. Tendonitis is most common in younger (<40 year) patients, whereas older individuals are more subject to full-thickness tears.
  - **Clinical Symptoms:** Acute or chronic pain. Loss of motion, RC weakness, disruption of sleep, and abnormal scapulothoracic motion are also associated symptoms.
  - **Radiographs:** Routine radiographs may be normal, or may show evidence of AC or glenohumeral arthritis, bone spurs, or calcific tendonitis. MRI is the "gold standard" and is indicated after failure of initial treatment or tear is suspected.
  - **Treatment:** A conservative trial of ice, rest, and NSAIDs are indicated early. It is recommended that larger tears in younger patients are treated surgically. Physical therapy should be instituted to restore strength, ROM, and scapulothoracic motion with particular emphasis on the scapular stabilizers. Arthroscopic repair will be required in treatment failures.

- ■ **Scapular Fracture**
  - **Definition:** Fractures involving the body of the scapula, scapular neck, scapular spine, glenoid, the acromion, and/or coracoid process.
  - **Mechanism of Injury:** Usually involves a fall or high-energy impact. Commonly seen in high-impact sports. Often seen in conjunction with other injuries: rib fractures, pneumothorax, pulmonary contusion, spine or head injuries.
  - **Clinical Symptoms:** Painful to palpation or ROM of the arm or back of the shoulder.
  - **Radiographs:** AP and trans-scapular lateral views are recommended. CT scan may be necessary to determine the extent of the fracture.
  - **Treatment:** Most non-displaced fractures can heal with sling immobilization, ice, and anti-inflammatory or narcotic pain medication with early ROM exercises to prevent stiffness. Displaced or unstable fractures require surgical treatment. Observation for pulmonary contusions should be considered.

- ■ **Sternoclavicular Sprains**
  - **Definition:** Spraining or tearing of costoclavicular and/or sternoclavicular ligaments. May include physical injuries in young patients.
  - **Mechanism of Injury:**
    - *Anterior:* Indirect force to the lateral shoulder, as in a fall to one side and a force of top of opposite shoulder.
    - *Posterior:* Direct force to anteromedial clavicle.

- **Clinical Symptoms**:
  - *Anterior*: Prominence of SC joint with swelling and tenderness.
  - *Posterior*: Proximal clavicle behind sternum.
    - It is a *medical emergency* when there is respiratory distress due to obstruction, vascular compromise with pulselessness, swelling or discoloration, pain, dysphagia or hoarseness.
- **Radiographs**: Apical or lordotic view. CT scan.
- **Treatment**:
  - *Mild*: Ice, sling, rest.
  - *Anterior*: Figure-of-8 brace, sling, NSAIDs.
  - *Posterior*: Reduce as soon as possible with posterior pressure on anterolateral shoulders, or if unreduceable, transport to hospital for definitive care.

■ **Thoracic Outlet Syndrome (TOS)**
- **Definition:** TOS involves compression of the subclavian vessels and/or the brachial plexus in the region between the intervertebral foramen, the first rib and axillae. Women are affected more often than men (4:1).
- **Mechanism of Injury:** Etiology is individualized but may be due to a congenital cervical rib, fibrous bands or fibrosis of the scalene muscles.
- **Clinical Symptoms**: May involve 1) arterial compression (arm or hand feels cold, becomes numb or fatigued with motion); 2) venous compression (discoloration or swelling of the arm after exercise); or 3) neural compression (pain or paresthesias or sense of heaviness). The following tests may aid the diagnosis: Adson maneuver and Roos test.
- **Radiographs:** Cervical spine radiographs, MRI, EMG, or nerve conduction studies may be indicated in the individual workup.
- **Treatment:** Correction of posture and stretching of the scalene and pectoral muscles, while strengthening the shoulder girdle musculature, aids in up to 90% of cases. Surgical treatment for cervical rib excision may be indicated.

PROCEDURES

■ **Acromioclavicular Joint Injection**
- **Indications:** Degenerative AC joint, trauma, overuse.
- **Patient Position:** Seated with arm hanging by side.
- **Technique:** Find lateral edge of acromion, move medially about thumb's width to find joint. Insert needle medially at about 30° angle to 3/8 to ½ inch depth.
- **Medicine/Needle:** 0.5 mL steroid/0.5 mL anesthetic/25 gauge.

■ **Glenohumeral Dislocation Reduction (Anterior >95%)**
- **Acute/On-field Approach:** Manipulation in slight abduction, forward flexion, and gentle internal rotation.
- **Stimson Method:** Patient lies prone on table with affected arm over the side. Hang a 5 to 10 lb weight freely from the wrist. Spontaneous reduction as shoulder muscles relax.

- **Scapula Manipulation**: Patient lies prone with arm flexed hanging off table. Rotate scapula medially by pushing on inferior tip and rotating the superior aspect of the scapula outward.

■ **Glenohumeral Injection**
- **Indications**: Arthritis, RC tendonitis, adhesive capsulitis.
- **Patient Position**: Seated with affected arm in relaxed position.
- **Technique**: Anterior approach. Arm held at side with elbow touching flank and forearm placed in external rotation. Identify crease between mechal border of anterior deltoid and lateral border of pectorals. Needle inserted into crease while arm internally rotated. Needle will be introduced into joint.
- **Medicine/Needle**: 1 mL steroid/6-10 mL of anesthestics/22-25gauge 1.5 inch.

■ **Subacromial Injection**
- **Indications**: Subacromial impingement syndrome.
- **Patient Position**: Seated with affected arm in relaxed position.
- **Technique**: Palpate lateral edge of acromion. Insert needle just inferior to mid-point of acromion and angle slightly cephalad.
- **Medicine/Needle**: 1 mL steroid/6-10 mL of anesthestics/22-25gauge 1.5 inch.

ELBOW INJURIES

HARD TISSUE (BONY INJURIES)

■ **Capitellar Osteochondritis Dissecans**
- **Definition**: Injury typically occurs in young athletes, with open growth plates, with damage to the articular surface of capitellum.
- **Mechanism of Injury**: Lateral compression forces mostly due to throwing. Also common in gymnastics.
- **Clinical Symptoms**: Pain with activity, loss of full extension, localized lateral swelling, and crepitation with motion. Improves with rest.
- **Radiographs**: AP and lateral radiographs may show loose bodies, irregularity, or capitellar flattening. MRI may be necessary.
- **Treatment**: Rest for several months. If loose bodies are present, surgical excision or debridement is indicated.

■ **Distal Humerus/Supracondylar Fracture**
- **Definition**: Distal humeral fractures make up only 2% of adult fractures but are associated with significant morbidity. The fracture should be closely evaluated to determine if the injury is displaced, comminuted, intra-articular, or if neurovascular structures are involved.
- **Mechanism of Injury**: Fall on the outstretched hand or point of the elbow.

- **Clinical Symptoms:** Swelling, deformity, ecchymosis, pain and reduction in the ROM are all symptoms.
- **Radiographs:** AP and lateral radiographs. Look for a possible fat pad or sail sign.
- **Treatment:** Non-displaced fractures may be treated conservatively with splinting for 7 to 10 days followed by protected ROM. Displaced, comminuted and intra-articular fractures often require open reduction and internal fixation surgical treatment.

■ **Elbow Dislocation**
- **Definition:** Elbows dislocate posteriorly 80% of the time. May occur with concomitant soft tissue injuries [e.g., UCL (ulnar collateral ligament) tear] or fractures [medial epicondyle (children) or radial head (adults)]. Most common dislocated joint in children.
- **Mechanism of Injury:** FOOSH.
- **Clinical Symptoms:** Pain, swelling, obvious deformity, and inability to bend the elbow. Examine neurovascular structures for associated injury.
- **Radiographs:** AP and lateral radiographs.
- **Treatment:** Reduction should be performed as soon as possible examining neurovascular status before and after reduction. Splint application and follow-up with AP and lateral radiographs are necessary to confirm a successful reduction. Early motion should begin within one week. NSAIDs or pain medication is indicated as necessary.

■ **Olecranon Fracture**
- **Definition:** Proximal ulna and posterior prominence of the elbow. Displacement and/or comminution of the fracture site are important to determine proper treatment.
- **Mechanism of Injury:** Fall on the outstretched hand or point of the elbow.
- **Clinical Symptoms:** Swelling and palpable deformity with occasional numbness of the 4th and 5th fingers secondary to swelling around the ulnar nerve or damage secondary to a comminuted fracture.
- **Radiographs:** AP and lateral radiographs. A true lateral is essential to evaluate the extent of the fracture and the articular surface.
- **Treatment:** Non-displaced fractures can be treated with a posterior splint or LAC with the elbow in 45° of flexion. Displaced or unstable fractures require open reduction and internal fixation. Follow-up films in 5 to 7 days are necessary to rule out fracture displacement.

■ **Radiocapitellar Chondromalacia**
- **Definition:** Compression force on radial side of elbow involving the radial head and capitellum causing osteochondral damage and possible loose bodies.
- **Mechanism of Injury:** Valgus overload, which causes repeated compression forces on radial elbow.
- **Clinical Symptoms:** Pain, catching and locking on lateral side of elbow.
- **Radiographs:** AP and lateral radiographs may reveal osteophytes, loose bodies, and loss of radiocapitellar joint space.

- **Treatment:** Acute injuries may be treated with rest, activity modification and correction of throwing mechanics. Chronic injuries, after joint damage has occurred, require surgical debridement. Recovery time depends on the amount of articular damage.

■ **Radial Head Fracture**
- **Definition:** Radial head fractures are classified as three types:
  - *Type I:* Non-displaced or minimally displaced fracture
  - *Type II:* 2 mm or more displacement of the radial head or angulation of the radial neck
  - *Type III:* comminuted fractures of the radial head and neck
- **Mechanism of Injury:** FOOSH.
- **Clinical Symptoms:** Pain, joint effusion and loss of elbow motion suggest a radial head fracture.
- **Radiographs:** AP and lateral radiographs are indicated. Look for a possible fat pad or sail sign.
- **Treatment:** Type I non-displaced fractures can be treated with a sling and/or posterior splint with early ROM when pain subsides. Aspiration of any hematoma with early ROM may be indicated for Type II injuries if the injury involves less than 30% of the joint surface. Severe Type II and all Type III injuries should involve surgical management.

SOFT TISSUE

■ **Distal Biceps Tendon Rupture**
- **Definition:** Distal bicep tendon ruptures are rare, involving only 3% of bicep ruptures with the remaining 97% involved at the proximal end. Rupture occurs at the radial insertion (radial tuberosity) and may be incomplete or complete. Injuries occur primarily in males >40 years of age.
- **Mechanism of Injury:** Extension force on a flexed elbow.
- **Clinical Symptoms:** Sharp, sudden pain in the antecubital fossa accompanied by weakness of elbow flexion and supination.
- **Radiographs:** AP and lateral radiographs are usually normal but may reveal an avulsion of the radial tuberosity. MRI is often indicated to define the extent of the tear.
- **Treatment:** Non-operative management is often sufficient for partial tears or in older patients. Modification of activity, splinting, ice, NSAIDs with eventual progressive strengthening is indicated. For complete tears in younger patients, repair of the bicep tendon to the radial tuberosity is indicated.

■ **Medial and Lateral Epicondylitis**
- **Definition:** Tension overload of the epicondyle attachment of the forearm and wrist flexors (medial) or extensors (lateral). Lateral epicondylitis ("tennis elbow") is 10 times more common than medial epicondylitis ("golfer's elbow").
- **Mechanism of Injury:** Repetitive stress causes microtears of the tendinous insertion at the medial or lateral epicondyle.

- **Clinical Symptoms:** Aching pain with active resistance.
- **Radiographs:** AP and lateral radiographs are usually negative, but may reveal calcific deposits.
- **Treatment:** Non-surgical management involves rest, ice, NSAIDs, counterforce bracing, stretching, eccentric strengthening, physical therapy modalities and correction of faulty mechanics in racquet sports. Corticosteroid injection may aid the resolution. If refractory to the above treatment, surgical debridement is indicated.

■ **"Nursemaid's Elbow"**
- **Definition:** Subluxation of radial head. Occurs in young children and is the most common elbow injury in children <5 years old.
- **Mechanism of Injury:** Occurs from a pull on the forearm when the elbow is extended and the forearm is pronated.
- **Clinical Symptoms:** Pain; child will not move elbow.
- **Radiographs:** AP and lateral films are usually normal.
- **Treatment:** Reduction by applying anterior pressure over the radial head, followed by supination of the wrist and elbow flexion.

■ **Olecranon Bursitis**
- **Definition:** The olecranon bursa is on the extensor side of the elbow over the olecranon process. Bursitis can occur due to inflammation, infection or trauma.
- **Mechanism of Injury:** Repetitive stress or a direct blow to the posterior elbow.
- **Clinical Symptoms:** Variable swelling over the tip of the elbow which limits motion and is often accompanied by pain.
- **Radiographs:** AP and lateral radiographs may be indicated depending on the clinical presentation.
- **Treatment:** If the swelling is minimal, treatment with NSAIDs, ice, and a compression wrap may be sufficient. If the swelling is significant, aspiration may be both diagnostic and therapeutic. If infection is suspected, aspiration with Gram stain, culture, and antibiotic treatment is indicated. Corticosteroid injection may be considered if there is no sign of infection.

■ **Radial Tunnel Syndrome**
- **Definition:** Posterior interosseous branch of the radial nerve becomes entrapped distally in the supinator muscle or proximally under the arcade of Frosche.
- **Mechanism of Injury:** Compression of the posterior interosseous nerve with repetitive overuse.
- **Clinical Symptoms:** Lateral elbow pain with pronation and supination motion accompanied by wrist extension and third finger extensor weakness. Positive Tinel sign distal to the lateral epicondyle. No sensory loss. May be misdiagnosed with lateral epicondylitis.
- **Radiographs:** AP and lateral radiographs are normal.
- **Treatment:** Rest, activity modifications and wrist extensor stretches. If recalcitrant, surgical decompression may be indicated.

■ **Ulnar Collateral Ligament Tear**
- **Definition:** Rupture or tear of the UCL (ulnar collateral ligament) over the humeroulnar joint.
- **Mechanism of Injury:** Valgus extension overload or repetitive valgus stress.
- **Clinical Symptoms:** Pain, tenderness, or joint opening with valgus stress at 30° of flexion. Loss of velocity with pitching or throwing.
- **Radiographs:** AP and lateral radiographs may be normal or reveal heterotopic spurring over the UCL or sublime tubercle of the ulna. MRI with contrast is indicated to determine the extent of the tear.
- **Treatment:** Non-surgical management is indicated for non-pitchers. This includes rest, ice, NSAIDs, and correction of throwing mechanics. For complete tears in competitive throwers, surgical reconstruction is indicated.

■ **Ulnar Neuritis (Cubital Tunnel Syndrome)**
- **Definition:** Compression of the ulnar nerve occurs most commonly in the "cubital tunnel" where it tracts between the head of the ulna and the distal medial humerus.
- **Mechanism of Injury:** May occur from a direct blow or leaning on the elbow for long periods of time.
- **Clinical Symptoms:** Numbness and tingling of the ring and little fingers with occasional pain at the elbow. Positive Tinel sign at the medial elbow.
- **Radiographs:** AP and lateral radiographs are usually normal. EMG/NCV studies may be indicated.
- **Treatment:** Activity modification and elbow bracing may allow the nerve compression to resolve. Surgical decompression and ulnar nerve transposition are indicated, if non-operative measures fail.

PROCEDURES

■ **Aspiration of Olecranon Bursae**
Sterile procedures should be instituted with the use of latex gloves and prepping the skin with a bactericidal solution. After infiltrating the skin over the bursae with 1% lidocaine, an18-gauge needle is used to aspirate the bursae. If clinical signs of infection are not present, a corticosteroid may be injected into the bursal cavity.

■ **Injection for Medial or Lateral Epicondylitis**
Sterile procedures should be instituted with the use of latex gloves and prepping the skin with a bactericidal solution. After infiltrating the skin with 1% lidocaine a 25-gauge needle is used to inject lidocaine and/or Marcaine into the irritated tendon. This is followed by a corticosteroid medication. Ice may be used after the injection.

■ **Reduction of Elbow Dislocation**
Reduction should be accomplished as soon as possible. Injecting the hemarthrosis with 10 cc of 1% lidocaine or the use of conscious sedation may make the

reduction less painful. Flexion of the elbow makes the reduction more difficult by lengthening the triceps attachment. Holding the elbow in a relatively extended position while performing in-line forearm traction and stabilizing the humerus results in a satisfying reduction. Supine positioning with elbow flexed off the table may make reduction easier. The elbow should be splinted in elbow flexion and post-reduction radiographs must be obtained to verify a successful reduction.

HAND AND WRIST INJURIES

FLEXOR TENDON

- ■ **Flexor Digitorum Profundus Tendon Avulsion (Jersey Finger)**
  - **Definition:** Avulsion of the FDP at its insertion of the distal phalanx.
  - **Mechanism of Injury:** Grasping of an object with forced DIP extension of the fingers during maximal FDP contraction. Commonly seen in football or rugby.
  - **Clinical Symptoms:** Inability to actively flex the distal interphalangeal joint. Flexion of the proximal interphalangeal joint is unaffected because the flexor digitorum superficialis is intact. The ring finger is most commonly affected because the FDP is usually weakest at that finger.
    - ◦ *Type I*: Tendon retracts to the palm
    - ◦ *Type II*: Tendon retracts to the PIP level
    - ◦ *Type III*: Bony avulsion
  - **Radiographs:** PA, oblique, and lateral views are indicated to evaluate for bony avulsion. Radiographs are usually negative.
  - **Treatment:** Varies depending on the type:
    - ◦ *Type I*: Surgical reinsertion within 7 to 10 days.
    - ◦ *Type II*: Early surgical repair within days, but no more than 3 to 6 weeks. May convert later to a Type I.
    - ◦ *Type III*: Operative repair, but can be delayed. May RTP with mitten-type splint, but no active gripping activities for 10 to 12 weeks post repair.
- ■ **Trigger Finger**
  - **Definition:** Pain in palm with digit locking and catching of digit.
  - **Mechanism of Injury:** Inflammation of flexor tendon sheath from chronic degenerative changes or acute pressure from bats, racquets, or golf clubs impeding normal tendon movement through flexor pulleys. Most commonly occurs at the MC head (A1 pulley).
  - **Clinical Symptoms:** Patient has difficulty extending affected finger actively, but may be extended passively. Often associated with painful snapping. Tenderness over the distal palmar crease over the MC head.
  - **Radiographs:** Normal.
  - **Treatment:**
    - ◦ *Conservative*: Steroid injection along tendon sheath, NSAIDs and activity modification.
    - ◦ *Surgical*: Release of A1 pulley.

EXTENSOR TENDON

■ Boutonnière Deformity

- **Definition:** Rupture of the central slip of the extensor tendon, proximal to its insertion on the middle phalanx, allowing the proximal phalanx to protrude through the lateral bands of the extensor tendon causing flexion of the PIP and extension of the DIP.
- **Mechanism of Injury:** Forced flexion of the middle phalanx during active PIP joint extension or by palmar dislocation of the PIP joint.
- **Clinical Symptoms:** Pain and swelling at the PIP joint with inability to actively extend the PIP with hyperextension of the DIP. A boutonnière deformity may take 1 to 3 weeks to develop.
- **Radiographs:** PA, oblique, and lateral radiographs are indicated.
- **Treatment:**
  - *Conservative:* A static or dynamic extension splint for 6 to 8 weeks with PIP in full extension.
  - *Surgical:* Failed splinting.

■ Mallet Fracture

- **Definition:** DIP flexion deformity caused by loss of continuity of the extensor mechanism to the distal phalanx. The extensor mechanism injury can involve a bone fragment or tendon rupture.
- **Mechanism of Injury:** Forced flexion of the DIP joint. Sometimes referred to as "baseball finger" from a ball hitting the tip of the finger.
- **Clinical Symptoms:** Pain, swelling, and inability to actively extend the DIP joint
- **Radiographs:** AP and lateral views. May have no abnormality other than flexion of the DIP.
- **Treatment:** Splint DIP joint in extension for 6 to 8 weeks. Surgical consult for bony fragments involving >30% of the joint surface or for tendon rupture.

■ Swan Neck Deformity

- **Definition:** Finger deformity resulting in PIP hyperextension and DIP flexion.
- **Mechanism of Injury:** Injury may occur at DIP, PIP, or MCP.
  - *DIP:* Mallet finger (rupture of terminal extensor tendon → stronger extension at PIP).
  - *PIP:* Distal volar capsule injury → lateral bands displace dorsally → stronger PIP extension and relaxation of DIP extension (especially with FDS rupture).
  - *MCP:* Volar subluxation and ulnar drift (rheumatoid arthritis) → muscle imbalances.
- **Clinical Symptoms:** Finger deformity.
- **Radiographs:** PA, oblique, and lateral radiographs are indicated.
- **Treatment:**
  - *Conservative:* Splinting with figure-of-8 or ring splint (slight flexion)
  - *Surgical:* Reconstruction to improve function

HARD TISSUE (BONY INJURIES)

■ **Distal Radius Fracture**
- **Definition:** Represents approximately 17% of all emergency department fractures. "Universal classification":
  - *Type I:* Nonarticular, nondisplaced
  - *Type II:* Nonarticular, displaced
  - *Type III:* Intra-articular, nondisplaced
  - *Type IV:* Intra-articular, displaced
    1) Reducible (stable)
    2) Reducible (unstable)
    3) Irreducible (unstable)
- **Mechanism of Injury:** FOOSH.
- **Clinical Symptoms:** Pain and restricted ROM with wrist flexion, extension, pronation and supination. Assess median nerve function.
- **Radiographs:** AP, lateral, and oblique views.
- **Treatment:** Most intra-articular fractures should be referred for consideration of surgical fixation. Nondisplaced fractures can be treated with a sugar tong splint for 3 to 4 days until swelling subsides and then cast immobilization.
  - *Nonarticular, nondisplaced or minimally displaced:* SAC for 3 to 6 weeks. LAC if significant pain with forearm supination/pronation.
  - *Nonarticular, displaced/angulated:* After adequate reduction, LAC for 3 to 4 weeks, followed by SAC for 2 to 3 weeks. Weekly radiographs to verify no reangulation.
  - *Intra-articular, nondisplaced:* LAC for 3 to 4 weeks followed by SAC for 2 to 3 weeks. Consideration for surgical consult for anatomic reduction.
  - *Intra-articular, displaced:* Surgical consult for anatomic reduction and ORIF.

■ **Distal Radius Fracture in Children (Torus or "Buckle" Fracture)**
- **Definition:** Softer bones in children "buckle" instead of break. Must not confuse with "greenstick" fracture (only involves one cortex), which may lead to a permanent bend unless fracture is completed.
- **Mechanism of Injury:** FOOSH.
- **Clinical Symptoms:** Pain and swelling at site of fracture.
- **Radiographs:** AP, lateral, and oblique views.
- **Treatment:**
  - *Buckle fracture:* SAC for 3 to 4 weeks and splint for 2 to 3 weeks for at-risk activities.
  - *Greenstick:* If angulated <10°, LAC in full supination for 3 to 4 weeks and SAC for 2 weeks with weekly radiographs. If angulated >10°, anatomic reduction and casting may be necessary.

■ **Fifth Metacarpal Neck Fracture (Boxer's Fracture)**
- **Definition:** Fracture of the 5th MC neck with dorsal angulation of the distal fragment. Accounts for 36% of all hand fractures.

- **Mechanism of Injury:** Direct blow, torsional or bending load to the hand. Typically results from a closed fist striking an object.
- **Clinical Symptoms:** Pain and swelling at the 5th finger. Visual loss of knuckle when making a fist.
- **Radiographs:** PA, lateral, and oblique views.
- **Treatment:** If angulation is greater than 40° to 50°, operative fixation is indicated. If less than 40° to 50°, closed reduction and casting in an ulnar gutter splint with the 4th and 5th finger MP joints flexed to 80° and the PIP and DIP joints extended provide optimal treatment.

■ **Hamate (Hook) Fracture**
- **Definition:** Hamate hook fractures account for 2% to 4% of all carpal fractures. The hook serves as the ulnar border of the carpal tunnel and the radial border of Guyon canal where the ulnar nerve travels. The hook also serves as the origin of the flexor and opponens digiti minimi muscles and functions as a pulley for the 4th and 5th finger superficial and deep flexor tendons.
- **Mechanism of Injury:** Injured by direct blow or shearing force. Dominant hand is affected in racquet sports while the non-dominant hand is affected in golf and baseball. May occur as a stress fracture.
- **Clinical Symptoms:** Tenderness to palpation over the hook with painful and weakened grip and pain with resisted 4th and 5th finger flexion. Because of the relatively poor vascular supply, fracture is prone to nonunion.
- **Radiographs:** AP, lateral, and oblique hand views are often negative. Carpal tunnel view is needed to image the fracture. CT is the gold standard for full evaluation.
- **Treatment:** Early diagnosis is crucial. Cast immobilization with 4th and 5th finger incorporation for 6 to 8 weeks is often successful if done within 7 days. Removal of the hook is indicated for late diagnosed fracture, displaced fractures, fractures involving nerve compression, or patients unwilling to be treated with prolonged immobilization.

■ **Kienbock Disease**
- **Definition:** Avascular necrosis of the carpal lunate.
- **Mechanism of Injury:** Trauma is suggested, but etiology is unclear.
- **Clinical Symptoms:** Wrist pain and stiffness.
- **Radiographs:** PA, oblique, and lateral views may be normal early on. Ulnar minus variant may be present. Tomography or bone scan may demonstrate abnormality. Future radiographs may show sclerosis, cyst formation, and carpal collapse.
- **Treatment:** Early treatment may revascularize lunate with ulnar lengthening. Arthrodesis or excision of the lunate may be indicated in later stages.

■ **Metacarpal Base Fracture**
- **Definition:** Fracture at the base of the MC, usually at the 5th or thumb MC.
- *Bennett fracture*: Intra-articular fracture at the base of the thumb.

- *Rolando fracture*: Intra-articular comminuted fracture at the base of the thumb.
- **Mechanism of Injury:** Striking a hard object.
- **Clinical Symptoms:** Pain and swelling at the base of the MC.
- **Radiographs:** PA, lateral, and oblique views.
- **Treatment:** Anatomic alignment is necessary, often requiring referral to a hand or orthopedic surgeon for consideration for ORIF.

■ **Metacarpal Shaft Fracture**
  - **Definition:** Fracture of MC shaft.
  - **Mechanism of Injury:** Striking a hard object with the fist.
  - **Clinical Symptoms:** Pain and swelling over the MC shaft. Complications involve shortening or malrotation of the fracture fragments.
  - **Radiographs:** PA, lateral, and oblique views.
  - **Treatment:** Nondisplaced fractures may be treated in a well-molded cast or orthosis for 4 to 6 weeks. Malrotation, displacement, or shortening more than 5 mm is unacceptable and difficult to maintain conservatively, requiring referral to a hand or orthopedic surgeon for ORIF.

■ **Scaphoid Fracture**
  - **Definition:** Most common carpal bone fracture. Estimated to occur in 1 of 100 college-level football players each year. May initially present as a sprain resulting in delayed diagnosis. Vascular supply to the scaphoid presents along the waist of the scaphoid. Proximal pole has no direct vascular supply.
  - **Mechanism of Injury:** FOOSH.
  - **Clinical Symptoms:** Pain in the anatomic snuff box. If initial radiographs are negative and clinical suspicion is present, immobilization is justified. A bone scan may provide a definitive diagnosis. Fractures may only be visualized after 72 hours.
  - **Radiographs:** PA view in neutral and with ulnar deviation, lateral view and closed fist view (scaphoid view).
  - **Treatment:**
    - *Nondisplaced fractures*: Treated with immobilization. Cast with slight palmar flexion and radial deviation. The literature suggests a LAC for 6 weeks followed by SAC for 4 to 6 weeks or until evidence of bone healing. Nonunion after 3 to 4 months may require bone grafting or electrical stimulation.
    - *Displaced fractures*: Fractures displaced more than 1 mm need accurate reduction, usually requiring ORIF.

■ **Scapholunate Instability**
  - **Definition:** Most common carpal instability pattern.
  - **Mechanism of Injury:** FOOSH.
  - **Clinical Symptoms:** Pain and swelling with persistent decreased grip strength, limited wrist ROM and point tenderness over the scapholunate interval. Delayed diagnosis secondary to presumption that injury is just a wrist sprain. Pain with Watson scaphoid shift test by placing thumb over

the distal pole of the scaphoid and moving the wrist in an ulnar or radial direction. Pain or a palpable clunk is felt.
- **Radiographs:** PA views show the scapholunate interval greater than 3 mm (Terry Thomas sign). The lateral view will show a scapholunate angle greater than 70° (normal is 30° to 60°). Clenched fist view will increase the scapholunate diastasis. MRI will demonstrate the extent of the injury.
- **Treatment:** Partial tears may be treated with cast immobilization. ORIF for acute avulsion injuries. Chronic injuries may require arthrodesis.

■ **Triquetral Fracture**
- **Definition:** Second most common carpal fracture in athletes.
- **Mechanism of Injury:** Falling on wrist with extreme dorsiflexion and ulnar deviation or bony avulsion via the strong dorsal capsular ligaments.
- **Clinical Symptoms:** Wrist pain, swelling, pain on palpation. Pain with wrist extension.
- **Radiographs:** PA and lateral films (best seen on the lateral view).
- **Treatment:** Immobilization for 3 to 4 weeks.

SOFT TISSUE

■ **Carpal Tunnel Syndrome**
- **Definition:** Entrapment or compression neuropathy of the medial nerve.
- **Mechanism of Injury:** Repetitive overuse is most common cause. Also occurs in pregnancy, thyroid dysfunction or any condition causing wrist edema.
- **Clinical Symptoms:** Pain, numbness and paresthesias of the median nerve distribution of the hand (thumb, index, long and radial side of the 4th finger). Clumsiness and night pain (due to sleeping with a flexed wrist) are common. Atrophy occurs with longstanding CTS. Symptoms relieved with wrist extension. Positive Tinel and/or Phalen signs.
- **Radiographs:** AP and lateral radiographs, if obtained, are usually normal.
- **Treatment:** Mild cases can be treated non-operatively with cock-up wrist splints during day and night, NSAIDs, ergonomic work modifications, and corticosteroid injection. Carpal tunnel release is indicated for those with positive EMG/NCV studies, atrophy, or failure of conservative methods.

■ **de Quervain Tenosynovitis**
- **Definition:** Inflammation or stenosis of the abductor pollicis longus or extensor pollicis brevis tendon sheaths on the radial side of the wrist.
- **Mechanism of Injury:** Repetitive overuse.
- **Clinical Symptoms:** Pain or swelling over the radial wrist aggravated by thumb extension. Positive Finkelstein test. Crepitation may be present of the APL or EPB.
- **Radiographs:** AP and lateral radiographs, if obtained, are usually normal.
- **Treatment:** Immobilization with thumb spica, NSAIDs, iontophoresis, or cortisone injection. Operative treatment is necessary if conservative methods fail.

■ **Dupuytren Contracture**
- **Definition:** Nodular thickening of the palmar fascia.
- **Mechanism of Injury:** Repetitive overuse. Has a genetic component in northern Europeans (Viking disease).
- **Clinical Symptoms:** Painless nodules in the distal palmar crease. Flexion of the fingers may result as the nodule thickens and contracts.
- **Radiographs:** Not indicated.
- **Treatment:** Splint may delay surgical treatment to excise the soft-tissue bands.

■ **Ganglion Cyst**
- **Definition:** A type of degenerative process of the joint capsule of the wrist forming a localized fusiform mass. The most common benign tumor of the hand and wrist.
- **Mechanism of Injury:** Typically no specific injury. May be associated with overuse. Often spontaneous in onset.
- **Clinical Symptoms:** May be asymptomatic or may cause pain. Pain can increase with activity.
- **Radiographs:** Usually unnecessary.
- **Treatment:** Observation if asymptomatic. May aspirate and inject corticosteroid. Surgical intervention if cyst persists or reoccurs.

■ **Guyon Tunnel Syndrome ("Cyclist's Palsy" or "Handlebar Palsy")**
- **Definition:** Ulnar nerve compression of the 4th and 5th finger.
- **Mechanism of Injury:** Compression or traction on the ulnar nerve in or near Guyon canal due to prolonged wrist hyperextension that occurs while riding.
- **Clinical Symptoms:** Numbness, tingling and/or weakness of the 4th and 5th fingers.
- **Radiographs:** Unnecessary.
- **Treatment:** Avoid wrist hyperextension by proper bicycle fit and handlebar padding, padded gloves, and frequent change in hand position while riding. May need surgical decompression if above treatments fail.

■ **Subungual Hematoma**
- **Definition:** Pooled collection of blood under the finger or toenail.
- **Mechanism of Injury:** Shearing force causes dyshesion of nail from nail plate
- **Clinical Symptoms:** May be bright red to dark brown depending on acuteness. May be asymptomatic or acutely painful.
- **Radiographs:** If suspicious of a underlying distal phalanx fracture, routine radiographs are indicated; otherwise not necessary.
- **Treatment:** If not painful, just observation. If painful, may use a 22-gauge needle and twist into nail until blood is expressed. Alternatively, use of a cautery or heated paper clip may also work.

■ **Triangular Fibrocartilage Tear**
- **Definition:** Ulnar side wrist pain due to acute or degenerative tear of the TFCC (**T**riangular **F**ibro**C**artilage **C**omplex). The TFCC has three functions:

1) primary stabilizer of the distal radioulnar joint; 2) transmits 20% of the load of the wrist; 3) supports the ulnar carpal bones.
- **Mechanism of Injury:** Usually due to wrist hyperextension, ulnar deviation, and axial load trauma or repetitive wrist injury.
- **Clinical Symptoms:** Loss of grip strength, ulnar side wrist pain, and pain with pronation, supination, and wrist extension. Pain on palpation between the extensor carpi ulnaris and flexor carpi ulnaris tendons in the soft spot distal to the ulnar styloid. Often there is pain or instability in the distal radioulnar joint.
- **Radiographs:** PA and lateral views are usually normal. MRI arthrography needed for diagnosis.
- **Treatment:** Conservative treatment includes immobilization for 6 to 8 weeks. Peripheral tears may heal secondary to good vascularity, whereas central tears may not heal, but be asymptomatic. Arthroscopy is indicated for those with ulnar side symptoms that preclude activities or who fail conservative treatment.

■ **Ulnar Collateral Ligament Sprain (Gamekeeper's or Skier's Thumb)**
- **Definition:** Tear or sprain of the ulnar collateral ligament of the thumb.
- **Mechanism of Injury:** Forced radial deviation of the thumb (i.e., fall on hand while gripping ski pole).
- **Clinical Symptoms:** Pain, swelling, and tenderness over the ulnar side of the MCP joint. Examination in full extension and at 30° of flexion with comparison to opposite side. Lack of firm endpoint or greater than 30° of laxity compared to contralateral side indicates injury. Important to distinguish partial versus complete tear. May need local anesthetic block to assist in diagnosis. A Stener lesion occurs when the ligament ends are displaced by the adductor aponeurosis.
- **Radiographs:** PA, oblique, and lateral views. MRI may assist to determine a complete tear or Stener lesion.
- **Treatment:** Partial tears will heal with cast immobilization for 4 to 6 weeks with the MCP in slight flexion. Complete tears require operative fixation.

PROCEDURES

■ **Carpal Tunnel Injection**
- **Indications:** Carpal tunnel syndrome.
- **Patient Position:** Palm up with wrist in mild extension.
- **Technique:** Insert needle just proximal to distal wrist crease at 45° angle just ulnar to palmaris longus tendon and angle toward index finger to depth of about ½ inch. May pop through transverse carpal ligament.
- **Medicine/Needle:** 0.5 mL steroid/0-0.5 mL anesthetic/25-27gauge

■ **de Quervain Tenosynovitis Injection**
- **Indications:** Overuse, inflammation of extensor pollicis brevis and abductor pollicis longus.
- **Patient Position:** Wrist in a vertical position with thumb flexed.

- **Technique:** Insert needle bevel up into sheath between tendons of EPB and AbdPL to about ¼ inch depth.
- **Medicine/Needle:** 0.25-0.5 mL steroid/0.5-0.75 mL anesthetic/ 25-27gauge

■ **Trigger Finger Injection**
- **Indications:** Trigger finger, stenosing tenosynovitis.
- **Patient Position:** Palm up.
- **Technique:** Insert needle just proximal to MP joint at distal palmar crease parallel with tendon toward fingertips to depth of about ¼ inch.
- **Medicine/Needle:** 0.25-0.5 mL steroid/0.5-0.75 mL anesthetic/ 25-27gauge

REDUCTIONS

■ **Distal Radius Fracture (Smith/Colle Fracture)**
Perform a hematoma block. Apply traction distally. Place thumbs on distal portion of fracture. Increase deformity through flexion/extension and realign by placing pressure on distal fracture. May be facilitated by having an assistant provide counter traction (above the elbow). Post-reduction radiograph mandatory for evaluation of fracture alignment.

■ **Finger Dislocation**
For reduction of a dorsal PIP joint dislocation, hyperextend the distal portion to "unlock" the joint and gently apply distal traction to the injured finger while applying volarly directed pressure to the middle phalanx.

HIP AND PELVIS

■ **Athletic Pubalgia ("Sports Hernia")**
- **Definition:** Syndrome of chronic, exertional pain at the tendinous insertion of the lateral rectus abdominus from a tear or attenuation of the rectus at the insertion at the pubic bone; pain can be debilitating and put an athletic career at risk.
The term "sports hernia" mischaracterizes the pathology.
  - More common in males.
  - Often associated with osteitis pubis.
  - Often seen in sports requiring vigorous rotational movement (hockey, soccer, football) but can been seen in all sports.
  - Often associated with strain or tear of hip adductors on inferior surface of pubic symphysis.
  - Diagnosis can be elusive: must rule out GI, GU, hip pathology and true inguinal hernia.
- **Clinical Symptoms:** Athletes present with groin pain exacerbated by activity. Examination reveals absence of hernia with tenderness worsened with resisted sit-up; tenderness at the distal rectus lateral to midline. May also have secondary pain near the adductor insertion sites onto the pubis.

- **Tests:** MRI may reveal muscle attenuation, "secondary cleft sign" or inflammation; can also identify or rule out other pathology.
- **Treatment:** Surgical if not improving with conservative methods (e.g., rest, core strengthening, corticosteriod injection).

■ **Avulsion Fracture of the Hip and Pelvis**
- **Definition:** Fracture of the ischial tuberosity apophysis where the above muscles attach. Occurs most commonly in skeletally immature athletes (i.e., Tanner stage 3).
- **Mechanism of Injury:** Sudden contraction or stretch of the muscles that attach to the apophysis.
- **Clinical Symptoms:** Sudden onset of pain and swelling, commonly with a "pop" of the involved muscle, associated with restricted ROM and strength.
- **Radiographs:** Comparative radiographs of the affected and uninvolved sides confirm the diagnosis.
- **Treatment:** Conservative measures with rest, ice, NSAIDs, and progressive strengthening. Surgical considerations for avulsed fragments greater than 2 cm in size.

■ **Bursitis**
- **Definition:** Bursae are fluid-filled sacs that lubricate points of friction.
- **Mechanism of Injury:** An inflammatory reaction occurs from trauma to the area or repetitive overuse. Common areas in the hip are: trochanteric (over the greater trochanter), ischial (over the ischial tuberosity), and iliopectineal (posterior to the inguinal ligament and between the iliopsoas muscle and the pelvis leading to anterior hip pain).
- **Clinical Symptoms:** Pain with movement or sitting.
- **Radiographs:** Often obtained, but normal.
- **Treatment:** Ice, relative rest, stretching, NSAIDs and consideration of cortisone injection.

■ **Femoral Stress Fracture**
- **Definition:** Microfracture of the bone most commonly in the femoral neck or femoral shaft.
- **Mechanism of Injury:** Repetitive microtrauma to a bony area. Aggravated by rapid increase in training or hard training surface (e.g., sidewalks) and inadequate footwear. May be related to lower leg or foot intrinsic factors.
- **Clinical Symptoms:** Pain or tenderness to palpation or active or passive ROM with limited ROM. Antalgic gait and pain with standing or hopping on one leg.
- **Radiographs:** AP and lateral view may be negative within the first several weeks. If clinically suspicious, consider bone scan or MRI scan.
- **Treatment:** Initial treatment is non-weight bearing with the use of crutches. Cross-training and progressive return to sport continues after radiographic evidence of healing. Correction of biomechanical defects must be undertaken. Femoral neck stress fractures can be differentiated

into: tension side (superior cortex) or compression side (medial aspect). Tension side often requires ORIF, whereas compression side is often managed conservatively.

■ **Groin Strain**
  • **Definition:** Adductor muscle strain.
  • **Mechanism of Injury:** Forceful contraction or stretch of the adductor muscles.
  • **Clinical Symptoms:** Groin pain over the adductors worsens with passive abduction or active adduction of the thigh. Occasionally, a defect in the muscle with associated ecchymosis, swelling, and tenderness. Large differential diagnosis.
  • **Radiographs:** Pelvic views to rule out avulsion fracture.
  • **Treatment:** Ice, compression, crutches, NSAIDs. Gradual passive stretching and RTP when strength returns.

■ **Hip Apophysitis**
  • **Definition:** Inflammation of the apophysis where tendons attach to the various bony prominences.
  • **Mechanism of Injury:** Overuse and inflexibility in the young athlete.
  • **Clinical Symptoms:** Pain at the site of attachment aggravated by movement. Sites and muscle attachment and ages of apophyseal closure include:

Site	Muscle Attachment	Age (years)
Iliac crest	Abdominals	Males 16-20 Females 14-18
Ischial tuberosity	Hamstring	19-25
Anterior superior iliac spine	Sartorius	21-25
Anterior inferior iliac spine	Quadriceps	16-18
Lesser trochanter	Iliopsoas	16-18
Greater trochanter	Gluteus medius/minimus	16-18

  • **Radiographs:** May show avulsion fracture.
  • **Treatment:** Relative rest, ice, NSAIDs, cross training, flexibility exercises. Gradual return to activity.

■ **Myositis Ossificans**
  • **Definition:** Calcium deposition into a hematoma after a contusion or muscle tear. Most common in the anterior thigh.
  • **Mechanism of Injury:** Direct blow or muscle tear.
  • **Clinical Symptoms:** Firm mass within musculature after hematoma.

- **Radiographs:** AP and lateral radiographs of area may show early calcification within 3 to 4 weeks post-injury. Maturation of the calcification occurs over the next 3 to 6 months.
- **Treatment:** Rest and avoidance of further aggravation of the tissue. Pulsed US may be beneficial along with gentle stretching. NSAIDs (e.g., Indocin) may decrease heterotopic bone formation. Use of protective padding or bracing when ready to RTP. Surgery rarely indicated, but if chosen, perform only after maturation of the calcification after several months. Must differentiate from osteosarcoma.

■ **Osteitis Pubis**
- **Definition:** Inflammation of the symphysis pubis causing pain in the lower abdomen and pelvis and characterized by sclerosis and bony changes of the pubic symphysis. Often associated with athletic pubalgia.
- **Clinical Symptoms:** Abrupt or insidious pain localized over the symphysis that may radiate to the groin, medial thigh or abdomen.
- **Pain** is exacerbated by activity or lying on side; clicking or popping sensation may be felt.
- **Physical Exam:** Indicates tenderness to palpation directly over the pubis symphysis with bilateral compression of the greater trochanters; hip adductor weakness.
- **Radiographs:** AP films may show bony changes or sclerosis of the symphysis; bone scan, CT findings; MRI showing bone marrow edema.
- **Treatment:** Rest, condition improves with time, PT, manipulation, steroid injection; surgery rarely may be necessary.

■ **Piriformis Syndrome**
- **Definition:** The piriformis muscle is an external rotator of the hip. Patients complain of a dull achy pain in the central buttocks.
- **Mechanism of Injury:** Acute twisting or trauma, prolonged sitting or standing.
- **Clinical Symptoms:** Pain over the central buttocks region between the greater trochanter and the ischium with occasional radicular symptoms, if the sciatic nerve is impinged. May mimic discogenic disease. Pain reproduced and also relieved by stretching in internal rotation.
- **Radiographs:** Standing AP pelvis often negative.
- **Treatment:** Ice, stretching of the hip external rotators, NSAIDs, physical therapy modalities, and occasional cortisone injections.

■ **Femoral Acetabular Impingement**
- **Definition:** Restricted ROM of the femoral head in the acetabulum.
- **Mechanism of Injury:** Accumulation of excess bone around the femoral head and neck causing femoral retroversion and restricted motion. Damage occurs to the articular cartilage and labrum.
- **Clinical Symptoms:** Hip and groin pain. May present between ages 20 and 50 years. Worse with prolonged sitting or walking. May worsen with uphill walking.
- **Radiographs:** Supine AP pelvis and cross table lateral views. Reveals excess bone on the femoral neck.

- **Treatment:** Lifestyle modifications to decrease level of activity. Chronic condition that does not respond well to physical therapy or hip injections. Debridement, periacetablular osteotomy, or total hip replacement may be necessary.

■ **Strains (Hamstring and Quadriceps)**
  - **Definition:** Stretching of the muscle resulting in micro or macro tears of the muscle fibers.
  - **Mechanism of Injury:** Rapid deceleration on a stretched muscle or sudden contraction. Injury may be aggravated by muscle imbalance between the quadriceps and hamstrings, limited flexibility, inadequate warm-up or muscle fatigue. May feel or hear a "pop."
  - **Clinical Symptoms:** Pain with active or passive motion, swelling, ecchymosis, palpatory tenderness and possible muscle defect or gap.
  - **Radiographs:** AP and lateral views usually obtained but often normal.
  - **Treatment:** Ice, compression, crutch walking, and progressive ROM and strengthening as tolerated.

■ **Thigh Contusion**
  - **Definition:** Bruise or tear of musculature resulting in bleeding into the muscle belly.
  - **Mechanism of Injury:** Direct blow or forceful stretch.
  - **Clinical Symptoms:** Pain, swelling, ecchymosis, and restricted ROM.
  - **Radiographs:** Initial radiographs unnecessary. If pain persists, rule out myositis ossificans.
  - **Treatment:** Minimize initial hematoma by ice, compression and wrapping the knee in maximal flexion. Avoid aggravating modalities (e.g., heat, massage, US) until contusion stabilized. Gentle stretching and progressive strengthening as tolerated.

SKELETALLY IMMATURE ATHLETES

■ **Legg-Calve-Perthes Disease**
  - **Definition:** Medial hip pain in children ages 3 to 8 years. Male to female predominance 4:1. May be bilateral.
  - **Mechanism of Injury:** Etiology unclear, but may be related to interruption in blood supply to the femoral epiphysis.
  - **Clinical Symptoms:** Deep hip pain and limitation of ROM and positive log roll test.
  - **Radiographs:** AP and frog leg pelvic films show sclerosis of the epiphysis and collapse. Changes may not be evident on initial radiographs; therefore, clinical suspicion is paramount. MRI or bone scan may show evidence early in the course.
  - **Treatment:** Maintenance of femoral head and epiphysis is paramount with crutch walking, casting, bracing, or occasional osteotomy. Orthopedic referral.

■ **Slipped Capital Femoral Epiphysis (SCFE)**
- **Definition:** Hip pain in children 8 to 15 years. Earlier diagnosis improves prognosis. More common unilaterally.
- **Mechanism of Injury:** Medial or posterior slippage of the capital femoral epiphysis occurs from forces across the proximal femur. Related to rapid growth or obesity.
- **Clinical Symptoms:** Groin pain with radiation to hip, knee, or medial thigh. Usually has limp with limited hip internal/external rotation. Positive flexion rotation test (leg external rotation with hip flexion).
- **Radiographs:** AP and frog leg pelvic films show irregularity of the epiphysis and posterior or medial slippage of the epiphysis (i.e., ice cream falling off the cone).
- **Treatment:** Initial treatment is non-weight bearing with referral to orthopedic surgeon for consideration of ORIF to prevent further slippage.

PROCEDURES

■ **Ischial Bursae Aspiration**
- **Indications:** Ischial bursitis.
- **Patient Position:** Place patient in lateral decubitus position with affected side up, lower leg flexed, and upper leg extended.
- **Technique:** Identify ischial tuberosity prominence. Find area of tenderness, insert needle toward center of area until contact is made with bone and then withdraw slightly. Pepper bursal area.
- **Medicine/Needle:** 1 mL steroid/3-5 mL steroid/21-23gauge.

■ **Piriformis Injection**
- **Indications:** Piriformis syndrome.
- **Patient Position:** Patient lies in lateral recumbent position with the affected side up.
- **Technique:** Find point of maximal tenderness approximately midway between ischial tuberosity and greater trochanter. Insert needle at a 90° angle to a depth of approximately 1-½ inches.
- **Medicine/Needle:** 1-2 mL steroid/4-8 mL anesthetic/21-23gauge.

■ **Trochanteric Bursae Injection**
- **Indications:** Trochanteric bursitis.
- **Patient Position:** Place patient in lateral decubitus position with affected side up, lower leg flexed, and upper leg extended.
- **Technique:** Identify greater trochanteric prominence. Find area of tenderness, insert needle toward center of area until contact with is made with bone and then withdraw slightly. Pepper bursal area.
- **Medicine/Needle:** 1 mL steroid/3-5 mL anesthetic/21-23gauge

KNEE INJURIES

OVERVIEW

- **Effusion:** The timing and location of soft-tissue swelling or intra-articular effusion gives clues to the potential diagnosis.
  - *Intra-articular effusion:* Suggests injury to structures inside the joint.
    - *Early (within hours):* ACL tear, patellar dislocation/subluxation, osteochondral defect; growth plate fracture in adolescent.
    - *Late (next day):* Meniscal tears, synovitis.
  - *Extra-articular swelling:* Suggests injury to extra-articular structure: MCL tear; Bursitis (pre-, infra-, or suprapatellar; pes anserine).
- **Palpation:** Knowledge of surface anatomy, bony landmarks, and joint line tenderness.
- **Functional Tests:**
  - **Lachman:** Gold standard for ACL laxity. Anterior translation of the tibia on the femur.
  - *Grade I:* 0-5 mm of translation.
  - *Grade II:* 5-10 mm of translation.
  - *Grade III:* >10 mm of translation.
  - **Pivot Shift Test:** Confirmatory test for ACL laxity.
  - **Anterior Drawer:** Anterior translation of tibia on the femur.
  - **Posterior Drawer:** Gold standard for PCL laxity. Posterior translation of the tibia on the femur.
  - **Varus/Valgus Stress Test:** Tests laxity of collateral ligaments.
  - **McMurray Test:** Meniscal injury.
- **Age of Patient:**
  - **Child/Adolescent:** Growth plate fracture.
  - **Senior:** Osteoarthritis.
- **Radiographs:** AP, lateral, notch, sunrise, oblique.

HARD TISSUE (BONY INJURIES)

■ **Osteochondral Defect/Fracture**

- **Definition:** Fracture of the articular cartilage of the patella or medial or lateral femoral condyle.
- **Mechanism of Injury:** Shifting or pivoting sports resulting in instability or giving way.
- **Clinical Symptoms:** Often a "pop" with early marked swelling and pain. Catching or locking if loose body is present. Recurrent swelling with activity.
- **Radiographs:** AP, lateral, tunnel, and sunrise views may reveal a chondral defect. MRI indicated if there is clinical suspicion.
- **Treatment:** Orthopedic surgery referral for reattachment, excision of lesion or consideration of osteochondral allograft.

SOFT TISSUE

■ Anterior Cruciate Ligament Tear

- **Definition:** The anterior cruciate ligament (ACL) is the main knee-stabilizing ligament. It is made of two major bundles (posterolateral, anteromedial). May avulse tibial spine in younger patients.
- **Mechanism of Injury:** Most common mechanism is non-contact with deceleration on the planted foot. May also occur with hyperextension force or combination of varus/internal rotation or valgus/external rotation.
- **Clinical Symptoms:** Often a loud "pop" associated with a rapid and large hemarthrosis. Positive Lachman test, positive pivot shift test. Occasional positive anterior drawer sign, but not reliable. Moderate pain and marked instability with ambulation.
- **Radiographs:** AP, lateral, notch. Evaluate for tibial spine avulsion (young patients) or Segond fracture (chip/fracture/avulsion of the lateral capsule off of the tibia, which is pathognomonic for an ACL rupture). MRI may clarify diagnosis, show bone contusion or associated injuries.
- **Treatment:** Initially knee brace for comfort, ice, and crutches. Surgical management required for most active patients, usually after resolution of effusion, restoration of ROM and control of gait. Opinions differ as to surgical approach (patellar tendon, bone-tendon-bone, or hamstring autograft or allograft).

■ Lateral Collateral Ligament Tear

- **Definition:** Injury to the lateral (fibular) collateral ligament and/or lateral capsular ligament. Rarely an isolated injury.
- **Mechanism of Injury:** Varus or twisting injury. Sometimes with hyperextension or blow to anteriomedial tibia.
- **Clinical Symptoms:** Pain over the lateral ligament complex. Sense of giving way into hyperextension with standing, walking, or running backward.
- **Radiographs:** AP, lateral, and notch views. Arcuate sign demonstrates avulsion of proximal fibula with posterolateral ligament complex suggesting posterolateral instability. Lateral capsular sign demonstrates avulsion of midportion of lateral capsular ligament with avulsion fragment of proximal lateral tibia. Associated with ACL tears and indicates anterolateral instability.
- **Treatment:** Grades I, II, and III similar to MCL strains. PRICE, crutches, and functional rehabilitation for Grades I and II. Surgical consideration for Grade III because of associated injuries and instability.

■ Medial Collateral Ligament Tear

- **Definition:** Injury to the medial (tibial) collateral ligament and/or medial capsular ligament.
- **Mechanism of Injury:** Valgus stress applied to knee most often by a blow to the lateral knee.

- **Clinical Symptoms**: Point tenderness at any point along the MCL. Extra-articular swelling. Pain with valgus stress at 30° flexion.
  - *Grade I*: Stretching of MCL fibers without laxity, but with pain.
  - *Grade II*: Partial tear of MCL fibers with mild laxity on valgus stress test and firm endpoint.
  - *Grade III*: Complete disruption of MCL fibers with significant opening on valgus stress test, often minimal pain.
- **Radiographs**: AP, lateral, and notch views. Pellegrini–Stieda disease (calcification within the MCL) suggests old injury.
- **Treatment**: Initial treatment for all stages is ice, NSAIDs, immobilization, and activity modification.
  - *Grade I*: Functional progression of rehabilitation within 1 to 2 weeks post-injury.
  - *Grade II*: Immobilization and crutches until patient has control of gait. Progress to function rehabilitation as pain permits over the next 3 to 4 weeks.
  - *Grade III*: Same as Grade II, but progression to RTP is often >4 weeks. Functional brace for RTP initially. Surgical referral if accompanied with other associated injuries.

■ Meniscal Tear

- **Definition**: Injury to the medial or lateral semilunar cartilage of the knee. May be degenerative (horizontal cleavage) or traumatic (oblique, radial, longitudinal, horizontal, or bucket handle). Tears may be partial or full thickness. Surgical consideration is dependent on the location of the tear (periphery in the vascular zone or more central in the nonvascular zone) or if it is full thickness. Traumatic tears are more common in the medial meniscus because it is less mobile than the lateral meniscus.
- **Mechanism of Injury**:
  - *Traumatic Tears*: Often from a single, weight-bearing event associated with rotational or deceleration force. May be associated with intra-articular ligament injuries.
  - *Degenerative Tears*: Result from repetitive loaded weight-bearing and rotational forces.
- **Clinical Symptoms**: Joint line pain with limited ROM and mild swelling that usually occurs by the next day after injury (not immediate). Occasional locking (may be associated with a bucket handle tear or displaced fragment). Patients may report instability with giving way sensation or recurrent swelling with activity.
- **Radiographs**: AP, lateral, and notch views. MRI has 94% sensitivity rate.
- **Treatment**: Surgical management is dependent on the degree of symptoms. If recurrent instability and swelling with activity or associated ligamentous tears, arthroscopic evaluation and partial meniscectomy is indicated. Meniscal repairs are indicated in the peripheral vascular zone. Controversy exists in the proper treatment of the older athlete with meniscal tear and osteoarthritis.

■ **Posterior Cruciate Ligament Tear**
- **Definition:** Tear of the part or all of the two major bundles of the PCL (posteromedial or anterolateral). May not be appreciated initially due to limited disability.
- **Mechanism of Injury:** Direct force on fixed anterior tibia (i.e., dashboard injury), fall on flexed knee on the tibial tubercle or valgus/varus force in full extension.
- **Clinical Symptoms:** Moderate effusion, but less than with ACL. Sensation of femur sliding anterior on tibia with deceleration. Positive "sag" sign and positive posterior drawer. Must also test for posterolateral corner injury.
- **Radiographs:** AP and lateral views. Consider MRI.
- **Treatment:** For mild laxity, treat with PRICE, and functional bracing and rehabilitation. Significant laxity, consider surgical reconstruction.

EXTENSOR MECHANISM PROBLEMS

■ **Bursitis**
- **Definition:** Inflammation of the various bursae around the knee.
- **Mechanism of Injury:** Repetitive overuse or direct blow.
- **Clinical Symptoms:** Swelling, pain, and dysfunction in prepatellar region (prepatellar bursae), proximal medial tibia (pes anserine bursae), medial joint line (tibial collateral ligament bursae), above the patella (suprapatellar bursae), or below the patella (infrapatellar bursae).
- **Radiographs:** Usually not helpful.
- **Treatment:**
  - *Acute:* Ice, compression, padding, and NSAIDs.
  - *Chronic:* Physical therapy modalities, aspiration, and corticosteroid injection.

■ **Iliotibial Band Syndrome**
- **Definition:** Lateral side knee pain often present in long-distance runners.
- **Mechanism of Injury:** Pain occurs during a run as the iliotibial band snaps over the lateral femoral condyle at 30° of knee flexion. Pain occurs from irritation of the inner portion of the band, interposed bursae, or lateral femoral condyle periosteum. ITB tightness, limb length discrepancy, foot pronation, and prominent lateral femoral condyle are contributing factors.
- **Clinical Symptoms:** Pain or swelling over the lateral femoral condyle made worse by repeated knee flexion and extension. Pain made worse from running downhill and relieved by rest. Positive Noble compression test. Ober test suggestive of ITB tightness.
- **Radiographs:** Usually not helpful. MRI may indicate thickening of the ITB versus intra-articular pathology.
- **Treatment:** Ice, NSAIDs, ITB and hamstring stretching, and activity modification. Correction of mechanical abnormalities, physical therapy,

and foot orthotics and strengthening hip stabilizers are useful. Local corticosteroid injection to the iliotibial bursae may be helpful.

■ **Osgood-Schlatter Disease**
- **Definition:** Occurs in preadolescence and early adolescents (ages 8-13 in girls and 11-15 in boys). Described as an osteochondrosis occurring at the tibial tubercle apophysis.
- **Mechanism of Injury:** Repetitive microtrauma or overuse.
- **Clinical Symptoms:** Pain, tenderness and swelling at the tibial tubercle. May be bilateral and prevent activity.
- **Radiographs:** AP and lateral views demonstrate an enlarged or irregular tibial tuberosity. Occasional loose ossicles separate from the tuberosity and are present.
- **Treatment:** Ice, NSAIDs, activity modification and physical therapy modalities (i.e., iontophoresis). Occasional functional bracing or padding. VMO strengthening.

■ **Patellar Subluxation/Dislocation**
- **Definition:** Complete (dislocation) or partial (subluxation) lateral displacement of patella from femoral trochlea.
- **Mechanism of Injury:** Valgus stress often accompanied by a twisting maneuver and a strong quadriceps contraction. May be associated with increased Q-angle, VMO weakness, and VL hypertrophy.
- **Clinical Symptoms:** Acute injury, often with a "pop" and immediate pain. Rapid hemarthrosis and marked pain.
- **Radiographs:** AP, lateral, oblique, and sunrise views. Evaluate for avulsion fracture on medial edge of patella. May consider MRI.
- **Treatment:** If patella is still dislocated, knee extension and gentle pressure on lateral patellar edge usually allows reduction. Temporary immobilization with straight leg immobilizer as needed for symptoms. Functional patellar bracing and comprehensive rehabilitation, ice, NSAIDs, and complete rehab. Surgical treatment for failed conservative measures.

■ **Patellar Tendinosis, "Jumper's Knee"**
- **Definition:** Initially may present as a tendonitis with inflammation of the tendon at the inferior pole of the patella. Tendinosis suggests a more chronic, degenerative change in the tendon. Apophysitis of the inferior pole of the patella is common in young athletes and is referred as "Sinding/Larsen/Johannsen" syndrome.
- **Mechanism of Injury:** Overuse of the extensor mechanism of the knee such as in jumping.
- **Clinical Symptoms:** Pain and tenderness at the inferior pole of the patella and less commonly in the body of the patellar tendon.
- **Radiographs:** Routine knee films are usually normal, but occasionally some irregularity seen at the inferior pole of the patella.
- **Treatment:** Initially, RICE. Iontophoresis and other physical therapy have been of some benefit. Functional rehabilitation with eccentric strengthening. Occasional improvement with patellar strapping. ASTYM or GRASTON therapy may be beneficial, as may percutaneous tenotomy.

■ **Patello-Femoral Syndrome**
- **Definition:** Anterior knee pain most commonly from the patella not gliding correctly in the femoral groove during flexion/extension of the knee. Sometimes called "chondromalacia patella," a term that should be used only after confirmatory arthroscopic evidence of patella articular cartilage damage.
- **Mechanism of Injury:** Often due to overuse from malalignment of the extensor mechanism or quadriceps weakness.
- **Clinical Symptoms:** Vague anterior knee pain worse with sitting in knee flexion (positive "theatre sign") or ascending or descending stairs, which loads the extensor mechanism. Occasional swelling and patella crepitation. Physical exams demonstrate VMO weakness, lateral riding patella with active quadriceps contraction and periretinacular tenderness.
- **Radiographs:** AP, lateral, sunrise, or Merchant view, but may be normal.
- **Treatment:** Initially ice, NSAIDs, functional bracing, physical therapy, and activity modification. Primary treatment is VMO strengthening. May evaluate foot biomechanics and alignment of lower extremity. A minimum of 4-6 months of physical therapy should be performed before surgical consideration. Surgical options include lateral release or extensor mechanism realignment.

■ **Plica Syndrome**
- **Definition:** The plica is a synovial fold that attaches from the suprapatellar region to the anterior fat pad. It is a remnant of embryologic walls that divide the knee into different pouches. In some patients, it persists throughout life.
- **Mechanism of Injury:** Overuse with knee flexion/extension or direct trauma causes inflammation and thickening of the plica band leading to pain and disability.
- **Clinical Symptoms:** If the plica is thickened it may be palpated over the medial patellofemoral joint. Tenderness over the medial femoral condyle.
- **Radiographs:** Standard knee radiographs do not assist in the diagnosis.
- **Treatment:** Ice, NSAIDs, activity modification, and physical therapy modalities. Cortisone injection may be indicated. Surgery for recalcitrant cases.

■ **Popliteus Tendonitis**
- **Definition:** The popliteus travels from the lateral femoral condyle to the posterior proximal tibia.
- **Mechanism of Injury:** Overuse injury occurs in downhill runners or walkers. Foot pronation causes tibial external rotation and stresses the popliteus tendon.
- **Clinical Symptoms:** Insidious onset of posterior lateral knee pain. Pain in the posterior lateral corner of the knee reproduced in the figure-four position. Pain increased with resisted external rotation.
- **Radiographs:** Usually not helpful.
- **Treatment:** Rest, ice, NSAIDs, physical therapy modalities, stretching and orthotics, if indicated.

PROCEDURES

- ◼ **IT Band Injection**
  - **Indications:** Overuse/recalcitrant ITB syndrome.
  - **Patient Position:** Seated with knee supported or lateral decubitus.
  - **Technique:** Identify the point of maximal tenderness at lateral femoral condyle. Direct needle posteriorly and slightly medially to ¼ to 3/8 inch between lateral femoral condyle, and 1/3 inch inside the border of the ITB. If bone contact, withdraw slightly.
  - **Medicine/Needle:** 0.5 mL steroid/0.5-1.5 mL anesthetic/23-27 gauge.

- ◼ **Knee Aspiration/Injection (Intra-articular)**
  - **Indications:** Inflammatory/degenerative arthritis.
  - **Patient Position:** May have patient lying with knee in 10° to 15° of flexion (towel beneath knee) or seated with knee flexed at 90°.
  - **Technique:** The authors prefer the superior lateral patella approach. Find lateral joint line and then identify lateral/superior edge of patella; soft tissue area easily palpated just lateral to patella. Inject needle slightly posteriorly and cephalad to a depth of approximately 1 inch.
  - **Medicine/Needle:** 4-5 mL anesthetic/21-25 gauge with or without 1 mL steroid.

- ◼ **Pes Anserine Bursa Injection**
  - **Indications:** Overuse/pes anserine bursitis.
  - **Patient Position:** Seated or supine with knee flexed.
  - **Technique:** Identify pes by having patient flex knee against resistance. Follow combined tendons to insertion on medial tibia. Insert needle just lateral to point of maximal tenderness and angle postero-medial to about ¼ inch depth.
  - **Medicine/Needle:** 0.5 mL steroid/0.5-1.5 mL anesthetic/23-25 gauge.

- ◼ **Prepatella Bursa Aspiration**
  - **Indications:** Prepatellar bursitis.
  - **Patient Position:** Patient supine with knee in slight flexion. May prop knee on towel roll.
  - **Technique:** Bursa lies anterior and inferior to patella. Palpate swelling over the patella and bursa. Aspirate with an 18-gauge needle from lateral/medial approach at inferior-most aspect of swelling and drain. Option of inserting small amount of steroid post aspiration.
  - **Medicine/Needle:** 2-3 mL anesthetic/25 gauge with or without 1 mL steroid.

LOWER LEG INJURIES

- ◼ **Achilles Tendonitis**
  - **Definition:** Overuse repetitive stress on the Achilles tendon causing inflammation and chronic irritation. May occur at the peritenon (4-cm proximal to the calcaneal insertion) or at the insertion of the calcaneus.

- *Acute*: Inflammation of the peritenon.
- *Chronic*: Prolonged mucoid degeneration of the tendon substance, more properly known as *Achilles tendinosis*.
- **Mechanism of Injury**: Repetitive overuse. Exacerbated by running up hills, on hard surfaces, or cutting and jumping sports. Aggravated by increased training, tight shoes, and poor running biomechanics or foot structure.
- **Clinical Symptoms**: Pain on palpation either at the calcaneal insertion or 4-cm proximal, crepitation, or swelling. Tender nodules may form on the paratendon. May be aggravated by Haglund deformity. Limited and painful ROM.
- **Radiographs**: Lateral view may show ossification or spurring off the superior calcaneous.
- **Treatment**: Relative rest, ice, stretching and strengthening exercises, physical therapy (iontophoresis or phonophoresis), NSAIDs, extracorporeal shock wave therapy (ECSWT), correction of foot biomechanics, adjustments in training, and night splints. Walking-boot, AFOs, or casting may be used temporarily. Stretching and eccentric strengthening exercises are necessary for recovery. Corticosteroid injections should never be used. Surgical consideration for recalcitrant cases.

▨ Achilles Tendon Rupture

- **Definition**: Rupture of the Achilles tendon occurs 2 to 6 cm above the Achilles tendon insertion. *Epidemiology*: Males between 30 and 50 years old, left side more than right, associated with cortisone injection to the Achilles, repetitive exercise or acute eccentric stress.
- **Mechanism of Injury**: Acute rapid eccentric stress resulting in a "pop" or sense of getting hit in the calf.
- **Clinical Symptoms**: Acute pain, palpable defect in the tendon, weakness with plantar flexion, and positive Thompson test (absent plantar flexion).
- **Radiographs**: Unnecessary.
- **Treatment**: Treatment may be surgical or conservative. Both treatments require an aggressive stretching and strengthening program for full recovery.
- *Surgical*: Recommended for athletes because of the low risk of re-rupture.
- *Non-surgical*: Cast immobilization for 8 to 12 weeks.

▨ Compartment Syndrome of the Leg

- **Definition**: Intrinsic swelling leading to excessive pressure in an enclosed fascial compartment leading to compression of vascular or muscular structures. The lower leg consists of four compartments: anterior, lateral, superficial posterior, and deep posterior.
- **Mechanism of Injury**: May have an acute (traumatic) or chronic (overuse) cause.

- *Acute*: May have a bony, muscular, or vascular etiology that causes increased fluid and pressure in the fascial envelope. Most common in the anterior or lateral compartments.
- *Chronic*: Pain limits activity but resolves within 10 to 30 minutes post exercise.
- **Clinical Symptoms**:
  - *Acute*: Swelling and edema in lower leg compartment, pain to palpation and passive stretching. Parasthesias and loss of foot dorsiflexion.
  - *Chronic*: Symptoms similar to acute injury, but less severe.
- **Radiographs**: AP and lateral tibia/fibula films if trauma is suspected.
- **Treatment**: Compartment pressure monitoring is the gold standard. Normal resting pressure: 0 to 8 mm Hg. Positive tests include resting pressure >15 mm Hg; 1 minute post-exercise pressure greater than 30 mm Hg or 5 minute post-exercise >20 mm Hg.
  - *Acute*: Emergent fasciotomy when pressure >30 mm Hg.
  - *Chronic*: Activity modification, but if this fails fasciotomy is indicated.

■ **Medial Gastrocnemius Strain ("Tennis Leg")**
- **Definition**: Injury to the medial head of the gastrocnemius near the musculotendinous junction. Injury is most common in middle age athletes (35 to 45 years old) participating in racquet sports.
- **Mechanism of Injury**: Eccentric load when the foot is dorsiflexed and the knee is forcibly extended. Injury occurs in the gastrocnemius because of its action across both the knee and ankle.
- **Clinical Symptoms**: Pain, swelling, and ecchymosis. Defect rarely palpable. Antalgic gait.
- **Radiographs**: Unnecessary.
- **Treatment**: RICE protocol with compression sleeve. Consideration for night splint to stretch gastrocnemius. Active stretching and strengthening can be increased as pain allows.

■ **Medial Tibial Stress Syndrome (MTSS or "Shin Splints")**
- **Definition**: Pain at the posteromedial tibial border usually due to overuse activities. May progress to stress fracture.
- **Mechanism of Injury**: Periostitis of the posterior tibia insertional fascia affecting tibialis posterior, flexor digitorum longus, or gastrocsoleus muscle. Postulated mechanisms are lower leg muscle imbalance; rapid increase in intensity, duration or frequency of lower extremity training; foot pronation; improper footwear; or running on banked surfaces. MTSS comprises 15% of running injuries.
- **Clinical Symptoms**: Tenderness or pain along the involved posterior tibial shaft that occurs with activity, but is relieved by rest.
- **Radiographs**: AP and lateral radiographs are negative. If bony cortex irregularity is seen or bone scan is positive, suspect stress reaction or stress fracture. MRI may confirm periostitis.
- **Treatment**: Ice, rest, or activity modification, NSAIDs, correct foot alignment with new footwear or orthotics. May resume activity when pain

decreases and after lower extremity strengthening and correction of muscle imbalance.

■ **Peroneal Neuritis**
- **Definition:** Inflammation of the peroneal nerve.
- **Mechanism of Injury:** Direct trauma to the peroneal nerve near the fibula head.
- **Clinical Symptoms:** Numbness, parasthesia, or pain in distribution of the common peroneal nerve along the lateral side of the lower leg and foot. May be caused by icing the lateral knee after injury.
- **Radiographs:** AP and lateral view to evaluate for fibular head fracture.
- **Treatment:** Rest and activity modification. If persistent, consider EMG.

■ **Peroneal Tendonitis**
- **Definition:** Inflammation or crowding of the peroneal tendons or tendon sheath in the fibro-osseous canal.
- **Mechanism of Injury:** Usual cause is repetitive trauma. Direct trauma (i.e., ankle fracture) or chronic lateral ankle instability may also be causative. Knee malalignment or cavovarus foot may also be considered.
- **Clinical Symptoms:** Pain, swelling, limited ROM and decreased strength. Thickening of the tendons may be present.
- **Radiographs:** AP and lateral radiographs to rule out bony impingement.
- **Treatment:** Rest, ice, stretching, activity modification, NSAIDs, and orthotics with lateral heel wedge. Short-leg walking cast or immobilization for 3 to 4 weeks or steroid injection into the tendon sheath may be considered.

■ **Plantaris Tendon Rupture**
- **Definition:** Pencil-sized muscle tapering down to a fine tendon that runs beneath the gastrocnemius and soleus muscles and attaches to the Achilles tendon or the medial side of the tubercle of the calcaneus. Functionally insignificant. Absent in 7% to 10% of the population.
- **Diagnosis:** History of "snap" or "pop" or stinging in the calf while stepping off on that foot or changing directions.
  - Deep calf pain with mild swelling and ecchymosis may be present.
  - Neurovascular exam is normal.
  - Transient disability from tear and swelling from hemorrhage.
  - Rule out Achilles tendon rupture, partial tear of the gastrocnemius, or eventual compartment syndrome or DVT.
  - Imaging usually not preformed but MRI can differentiate injuries.
- **Treatment:** Elastic support (e.g., Ace wrap, TED stocking) from foot to tibial tuberosity. Heel elevation, RICE initially then heat after 24 hours. Analgesics as needed. May need crutches for several days; advance to weight bearing as comfort allows.
- **RTP:** Gradual return to activity as pain allows.

■ **Peroneal Tendon Subluxation**
- **Definition:** "Snapping" sensation over the lateral ankle with partial or complete rupture of the superior peroneal retinaculum.

- **Mechanism of Injury**: Sudden dorsiflexion with reflex contraction of the peroneal muscles. Sports participation responsible for 92% of injuries with skiing alone accounting for 66%.
- **Clinical Symptoms**: Swelling and painful "popping" sensation reproducible with dorsiflexion or foot eversion. Ankle stability tests are normal.
- **Radiographs**: AP, lateral, and mortise views are indicated.
- **Treatment**: Non-surgical management includes short leg casting for 4 to 6 weeks in slight plantar flexion and inversion followed by ROM and strengthening exercises. Surgical management is often employed for athletes with direct repair of the superior peroneal retinaculum.

■ Proximal Tibial-Fibular Joint Pain
- **Definition:** Pain due to inflammation or instability of the proximal tibia-fibular articulation.
- **Mechanism of Injury**: Usually due to a blow to the area.
- **Clinical Symptoms**: Pain to resisted dorsiflexion and eversion of the foot stressing the tibio-fibular joint. Positive Tinel sign over peroneal nerve. Popping or shifting at the joint.
- **Radiographs:** AP and lateral tib-fib films. MRI or CT scan may helpful.
- **Treatment:** Rest, ice, NSAIDs. Consider cortisone injection. Surgical stabilization for persistent cases.

■ Tibial Contusion
- **Definition:** Bruise that usually occurs in anterior or lateral compartment.
- **Mechanism of Injury**: Blow from a kick by an opponent's kick, stick, or ball.
- **Clinical Symptoms**: Pain, guarding, swelling, and antalgic gait. May lead to the following complications: compartment syndrome, subperiosteal hematoma, tibial or fibular fracture, or peroneal nerve palsy.
- **Radiographs:** AP and lateral films to evaluate for fracture.
- **Treatment:** Ice, elevation, compression, and NSAIDs. Limited weight-bearing or muscle contraction that may worsen injury. Relative rest until able to continue activity.

■ Tibial Stress Fracture
- **Definition:** Fatigue fracture of the posterior proximal or distal third of tibia. Most common stress injury in athletes. Progresses from MTSS to stress reaction to stress fracture.
- **Mechanism of Injury:** Insidious onset of pain associated with repetitive activities with the same mechanisms as in MTSS.
- **Clinical Symptoms:** Progressive posterior tibial pain initially occurring with activity that is not relieved by rest. Pain with palpation and percussion tenderness. Positive tuning fork test.
- **Radiographs:** AP and lateral views reveal periosteal reaction, thickened cortex or radiolucent line or "dreaded black line." Positive bone scan or MRI. MRI may reveal soft-tissue pathology.
- **Treatment:** Prolonged rest and avoidance of aggravating activity. Cross-training and immobilization until pain free. Correction of factors in MTSS. Consider tibial nail for refractory case.

HARD TISSUE (BONY INJURIES)

■ **Ankle Fracture**
  • **Definition:** Fractures of one or both of the malleoli or spiral fractures of the fibula. Two types:
    ○ *Stable fractures*, which do not involve the articular surface or disrupt the joint stability
    ○ *Unstable fractures*, which involve much of the articular surface and cause instability of the ankle joint
  • **Classifications:**
    ○ *Danis-Weber Classification:*
    ○ *Type A*: Fibular fracture below the syndesmosis
    ○ *Type B*: Fracture at the level of the syndesmosis
    ○ *Type C*: Fracture above the syndesmosis
  • *Lauge-Hansen Classification:* Based upon the mechanism of injury
  • **Mechanism of Injury:** Usually foot external rotation with either pronation or supination
  • **Clinical Symptoms:** Pain, inability to bear weight, deformity, bony tenderness. Crucial to evaluate neurovascular status prior to realignment.
  • **Radiographs:** AP, lateral and oblique internal rotation (mortise view).
  • **Treatment:** Open fractures require urgent irrigation and debridement followed by antibiotics. Displaced fractures require ORIF. Non-displaced with intact mortise can be treated with cast immobilization for 4 to 6 weeks and functional bracing and rehabilitation.

■ **Anterior Impingement**
  • **Definition:** Anterior ankle impingement may be bony or soft tissue.
  • **Mechanism of Injury:** Repetitive trauma to the anterior ankle capsule.
  • **Clinical Symptoms:** Persistent anterior ankle pain and loss of dorsiflexion after an ankle sprain. Soccer players, dancers, and runners are more susceptible. Persistent pain, catching, instability, swelling, gait alteration, or limitation of activity. Pain with forced plantar flexion, and pressure over the anterior lateral ankle and move the foot in forced dorsiflexion.
  • **Radiographs:** AP and lateral views. Consider dorsiflexion stress radiographs to evaluate anterior osteophytes on the tibia and talus. Consider MRI scan.
  • **Treatment:** Consider cortisone injection or surgical treatment for those who fail conservative measures.

■ **Calcaneal Apophysitis (Sever Disease)**
  • **Definition:** Heel pain in boys or girls (ages 8 to 13 years). May be unilateral or bilateral
  • **Mechanism of Injury:** May be related to overuse and microtrauma, heel cord or hamstring flexibility. May be traumatic. May be related to biomechanic abnormalities: pes planus or pes cavus, hallus valgus, or forefoot varus

- **Clinical Symptoms:** Pain on the posterior heel with tenderness to palpation or squeeze at Achilles insertion. Worse with standing on tip-toes.
- **Radiographs:** Usually normal; may see sclerosis or density at the apophysis.
- **Treatment:** Ice, heel lifts, Achilles stretching, NSAIDs. Consider orthotics or casting for severe pain.

■ **Haglund Syndrome**
- **Definition:** Protrusion of the posterior superior calcaneus.
- **Mechanism of Injury:** Recurrent stress from shoes with low heel counter. May appear similar to a "pump bump" but is bony tissue.
- **Clinical Symptoms:** Soft-tissue swelling at the Achilles tendon insertion. Pain on palpation.
- **Radiographs:** Lateral calcaneal view may reveal Haglund deformity.
- **Treatment:** Pad, ice, NSAIDs. Consider steroid injection or surgical treatment for those who fail conservative treatment.

■ **Os Trigonum Syndrome (OTS or Posterior Impingement Syndrome)**
- **Definition:** The os trigonum is an accessory ossicle on the posterior talus that occurs in approximately 23% of the general population.
- **Mechanism of Injury:** Repetitive trauma or a single event of forced plantarflexion. May involve a bony fracture of the ossicle or pain from the fibrous connection.
- **Clinical Symptoms:** Non-specific posterior ankle pain worsened with passive or active ankle plantarflexion. Negative "two-fingered squeeze" test that would be positive with retrocalcaneal bursitis.
- **Radiographs:** AP and lateral ankle views. Bony impingement may be evident on lateral view with maximal plantarflexion.
- **Treatment:** Activity modification, immobilization, or NSAIDs. Consider diagnostic injection with local anesthetic or treatment injection with cortisone. Surgical excision for recalcitrant cases.

■ **Talar Dome Osteochondral Lesion**
- **Definition:** Compression injury to the superior dome of the talus, usually involving the lateral talar dome.
- **Mechanism of Injury:** Inversion or eversion of the ankle. May be noted acutely, but may be a symptom of chronic pain after a "sprain."
- **Clinical Symptoms:** Ankle effusion and tenderness over the talus.
- **Radiographs:** AP, lateral, mortise, and plantarflexed mortise views. If clinical suspicion, order MRI or CT scan to aid in diagnosis.
- **Treatment:**
  - *Acute, non-displaced*: Immobilize in cast or rigid brace for 6 weeks, then ankle rehab.
  - *Acute or chronic displaced*: Surgical excision or fracture replacement and internal fixation. May require autologous osteochondral transplantation or drilling of the lesion.
  - *Chronic, non-displaced*: Surgical excision of the lesion. May have chronic symptoms.

SOFT TISSUE

- **Ankle (Lateral Inversion) Sprain**
  - **Definition:** Sudden pain of the lateral ligament structures resulting in pain and instability. 85% of all ligament injuries are lateral sprains.
  - **Mechanism of Injury:** Plantar flexion, inversion, and internal rotation result in tearing of the anterior talofibular, calcaneofibular, posterior talofibular ligaments, respectively. If the stress is severe enough, the medial malleolus may be avulsed or the distal fibular may be fractured.
  - **Clinical Symptoms:** Immediate swelling, ecchymosis, lateral tenderness, and pain with weight bearing.
  - **Radiographs:** AP, lateral, and mortise views.
  - **Treatment:** Ice, immobilization, NSAIDs, controlled ROM. Progressive stretching, strengthening and proprioception training. Early functional motion as tolerated. Taping and bracing for play.

- **Ankle (Medial Eversion) Sprain**
  - **Definition:** Damage to the medial structures of the ankle (deltoid ligament) make up 10% of ankle sprains.
  - **Mechanism of Injury:** External rotation, dorsiflexion, and pronation.
  - **Clinical Symptoms:** Symptoms similar to lateral ankle sprain
  - **Radiographs:** AP, lateral, and mortise views may show medial malleolar fractures or widening of the ankle mortise. May need stress views.
  - **Treatment:** Similar to lateral sprains, but medial sprains take longer to heal.

- **Anterior Tibialis Tendonitis**
  - **Definition:** The anterior tibialis accounts for 80% of ankle dorsiflexion strength. Tenosynovitis and rupture are possible.
  - **Mechanism of Injury:** Chronic overuse with running downhill or hiking. May be aggravated by shoelace pressure.
  - **Clinical Symptoms:** Pain and swelling over the anterior ankle. May mimic a compartment syndrome. Rupture, though uncommon, may lead to foot-drop.
  - **Radiographs:** Standard radiographs are not helpful.
  - **Treatment:** Tenosynovitis requires overuse modification treatment. Rupture requires surgical treatment.

- **Flexor Hallucis Tendonitis**
  - **Definition:** Irritation of the flexor hallucis tendonitis posterior to the medial malleolus
  - **Mechanism of Injury:** Overuse in runners and athletes involving repetitive stop and start or push-off activities.
  - **Clinical Symptoms:** Pain posterior to the medial malleolus with flexion of the great toe.
  - **Radiographs:** Standard radiographs are not helpful.
  - **Treatment:** Overuse treatments: ice, NSAIDs, activity modification, heel lift, rigid shoes or stiff shank.

- ■ **Peroneal Tendonitis/Subluxation**
  - **Definition:** The peroneus longus and brevis travel posterior to the distal aspect of the lateral malleolus covered by a soft tissue retinacular "roof."
  - **Mechanism of Injury:** Overuse of the tendon causes avascularity and irritation.
  - **Clinical Symptoms:** Pain with plantar flexion and inversion, along with active resisted dorsiflexion and eversion. Swelling may be present. The tendons may "snap" or sublux with active dorsiflexion and eversion.
  - **Radiographs:** Standard radiographs are not useful.
  - **Treatment:** Overuse treatments: ice, NSAIDs, activity modification. Eccentric strengthening. U-shaped felt pad with taping. Consider cortisone injection or cast immobilization. With failed conservative management for subluxing tendons, surgical treatment to restore the retinacular roof may be indicated.

- ■ **Posterior Tibial Tendonitis/Dysfunction**
  - **Definition:** The posterior tibial tendon stabilizes the longitudinal arch on its insertion at the navicular. Rupture is rare.
  - **Mechanism of Injury:** Chronic rubbing at the medial malleolus causes tendonitis and tenosynovitis.
  - **Clinical Symptoms:** Pain with active inversion and plantar flexion as well as single toe raise. Sometimes leads to foot hyperpronation and posterior tibialis dysfunction.
  - **Radiographs:** Standard radiographs are not useful. MRI if tear is suspected.
  - **Treatment:** Overuse treatments: ice, NSAIDs, rest with medial arch support or custom orthotics. Consider surgical treatment if evidence of a tear.

- ■ **Retro-Achilles Bursitis ("Pump Bump")**
  - **Definition:** Pain and swelling at the superior calcaneal tuberosity.
  - **Mechanism of Injury:** Poor-fitting shoes and development of lesion on posterior calcaneal.
  - **Clinical Symptoms:** Redness, swelling, and pain directly below the insertion of the Achilles tendon.
  - **Radiographs:** Standard radiographs are usually not helpful.
  - **Treatment:** Ice, massage, change shoe, or apply padding. Consider cortisone injection.

- ■ **Retrocalcaneal Bursitis**
  - **Definition:** Inflammation and thickening of the retrocalcaneal bursa located between the Achilles tendon insertion and calcaneus.
  - **Mechanism of Injury:** Overuse injury. May be caused by shoe heel counter being too constrictive.
  - **Clinical Symptoms:** Pain, swelling, tenderness anterior to Achilles insertion. Pain reproduced with palpation of the bursa with "two finger squeeze" test.

- **Radiographs:** Lateral view may show bone deposition on the posterior superior calcaneus (Haglund deformity).
- **Treatment:** Ice, NSAIDs, and correction of shoe wear. Cortisone injection into the bursa, but not into the Achilles tendon may be considered. Rarely, surgical debridement is necessary.

■ Syndesmosis Injuries

- **Definition:** Damage of the syndesmosis requiring a long course of rehabilitation. If no bony involvement, referred to as a "high ankle sprain."
- **Mechanism of Injury:** External rotation with forced dorsiflexion and abduction.
- **Clinical Symptoms:** Swelling and ecchymosis of the anterolateral ankle proximal to the joint. Tenderness to palpation over the anterior tibiofibular ligament. Often pain radiating to the proximal syndesmosis. If pain in proximal fibular suspect Maisonneuve fracture. Pain with passive external foot rotation with dorsiflexion.
- **Radiographs:** AP, lateral, and mortise views. Carefully examine for widening of the mortise. Diastasis is suspected with >4 mm of the tibiofibular clear space. Consider external rotation stress view or weight-bearing views.
- **Treatment:** Treatment is dependent on radiographic diastasis:
  - *Sprain without diastasis*: Stable injury. Weight bearing as tolerated with a high pneumatic brace or walking boot. If severe, consider immobilization up to 4 weeks. Patients should be warned of protracted recovery that is double the time for a lateral ankle sprain—often 6 to 8 weeks.
  - *Sprain with diastasis on stress radiographs*: If syndesmosis is anatomic and confirmed by CT or MRI, may be treated in non-weight-bearing cast or brace for 4 week and progressive weight bearing over the next 2 to 4 weeks.
  - *Frank diastasis with or without proximal fibula fracture*: Operative fixation with syndesmosis screws.
  - *Frank diastasis with Weber B or C fibular fracture*: Surgical fixation of ankle fracture with addition of syndesmosis screw.

PROCEDURES

■ Ankle Injection/Aspiration

- **Indications:** Soft tissue impingement, synovitis, chronic capsulitis.
- **Patient Position:** seated or supine, ankle slightly plantarflexed.
  - **Technique:** Identify small triangular hollow area just medial to the anterior tibial tendon. Located between medial malleoulus and the tibia talus articulation. Have assistant give gentle distraction to open up space. Insert needle into recess to depth of ½ to 1 inch.
- **Medicine/Needle:** 0.5-0.75 mL steroid/2-5 mL anesthetic/23-25 gauge.

■ Retrocalcaneal Bursa Injection

- **Indications:** Retrocalcaneal bursitis.
- **Patient Position:** Patient lies prone with foot in slight dorsiflexion.

- **Technique:** Identify superior edge of calcaneous. Insert needle from lateral position just superior to calcaneous and anterior to Achilles tendon.
- **Medicine/Needle:** 0.5 mL steroid/1.5 mL anesthetic/23 gauge.

FOOT INJURIES

HINDFOOT

■ **Calcaneal Stress Fracture**
- **Definition:** Overuse injury to the calcaneus.
- **Mechanism of Injury:** Sudden increase in exercise or runners who train on asphalt or concrete. Common in running or jumping sports.
- **Clinical Symptoms:** Sudden onset of pain. Percussion or palpation tenderness.
- **Radiographs:** AP and lateral view negative early. CT scan, bone scan, or MRI are necessary if clinical suspicion.
- **Treatment:** Non-weight-bearing with crutches for ambulation if cannot tolerate walking. Pool activities to maintain cardiovascular fitness.

■ **Plantar Fasciitis**
- **Definition:** Overload stress to plantar fascia causing microtears and inflammation.
- **Mechanism of Injury:** Tightness of gastrosoleus complex and heelcord along with foot pronation or pes cavus puts stress on the plantar fascia insertion at the calcaneus.
- **Clinical Symptoms:** Pain to palpation of the anterior medial calcaneus. Pain with first step in the morning (secondary to relaxation of the foot and shortening of the plantar fascia during sleep). Relieved by activity and recurs with rest.
- **Radiographs:** AP and lateral calcaneal view are usually negative. A traction spur may be seen, but is a result of the problem rather than the cause and is usually a late finding.
- **Treatment:** Ice massage, cross friction massage, heel lift, correction of foot biomechanics, night splints, taping, and NSAIDs are all employed. Stretching of heel cord and gastrocsoleus complex is required. Casting, cortisone injection, extracorporeal shock wave therapy, ASTYM or GRASTON and surgical release may be indicated for recalcitrant cases.

■ **Subtalar (Peritalar) Dislocation**
- **Definition:** Disruption of the talonavicular joint capsule with subluxation or dislocation of the subtalar joint.
- **Mechanism of Injury:** Traumatic rotational injury to the hindfoot with either forced inversion or eversion. With multiple ligament injuries the posterior tibial tendon and the articular cartilage may also be damaged.
- **Clinical Symptoms:** Obvious hindfoot deformity with protrusion of the talar head on either side of the ankle. Neurovascular structures must be examined.

- **Radiographs:** AP and lateral views. CT scan often indicated to evaluate occult injuries.
- **Treatment:** Reduction under anesthesia. Aggressive physical therapy after swelling and pain has diminished. Prognosis is guarded.

MIDFOOT

■ Compression Neuropathy ("Jogger's Foot")

- **Definition:** Entrapment of the medial plantar nerve distal to the tarsal tunnel.
- **Mechanism of Injury:** Overuse.
- **Clinical Symptoms:** Pain or numbness of the medial sole and medial toes.
- **Radiographs:** AP, lateral, and oblique foot films often negative.
- **Treatment:** Rest, NSAIDs, or soft orthoses. Steroid injection. Surgical release if failed non-operative management.

■ Cuboid Syndrome

- **Definition:** Lateral foot pain localized over the cuboid.
- **Mechanism of Injury:** Running on uneven ground or after lateral ankle sprain or lateral midfoot injury.
- **Clinical Symptoms:** Pain, weakness, or midfoot instability. Pain over the plantar aspect of the cuboid. Swelling may occur.
- **Radiographs:** Standard radiographs are usually negative.
- **Treatment:** Osteopathic manipulation (cuboid whip). Taping for sports participation.

■ Lisfranc Injuries

- **Definition:** Bony, ligamentous, or mixed injury involving the Lisfranc ligament that spans the second metatarsal base to the medial cuneiform.
- **Mechanism of Injury:** Forefoot hyperdorsiflexion or hyperplantarflexion.
- **Clinical Symptoms:** Midfoot pain and inability to bear weight, especially on tip-toes.
- **Radiographs:** AP, lateral and oblique foot films are often normal, especially in ligamentous injuries. Standing weight-bearing films with contralateral comparison demonstrates widening. The "clear space" should not exceed 2 mm. MRI can show ligaments well.
  - *Stage I:* No diastasis or loss of arch height.
  - *Stage II:* Diastasis of the I-II metatarsal bases is present with no loss of arch height.
  - *Stage III:* Diastasis of the I-II metatarsal bases is present with loss of arch height.
- **Treatment:** Treatment strategies are dependent on degree of diastasis. Many advocate rigid fixation for any degree of diastasis. Prolonged non-weight-bearing if conservative management is chosen. Any widening should be referred to a foot or ankle orthopedist.

■ **Morton Foot**
- **Definition:** The second toe is longer than the first with a short, hyper-mobile first ray.
- **Mechanism of Injury:** Hypermobility of the first ray leads to overpronation and increased load placed on the second metatarsal head.
- **Clinical Symptoms:** Callous under the second metatarsal head with midfoot pain.
- **Radiographs:** AP, lateral, and oblique views or show thickening of the second metatarsal or posterior displacement of the sesamoids.
- **Treatment:** Metatarsal pad proximal to the second metatarsal head. Medial heel wedge or arch support may also be indicated.

■ **Navicular Stress Fractures**
- **Definition:** Persistent pain on the medial midfoot aggravated by overuse activities.
- **Mechanism of Injury:** Overuse injury. Contributing factors are pes cavus and forefoot adductus.
- **Clinical Symptoms:** Midfoot or medial arch pain, but often difficult to pinpoint. Increased pain with weight-bearing.
- **Radiographs:** AP, lateral and oblique foot view often negative. If seen, the fracture is in central 1/3 of the bone. CT, bone scan, or MRI may be considered based upon clinical suspicion.
- **Treatment:**
  - *Conservative management for non-displaced and incomplete fracture:* 6 to 8 weeks of non-weight-bearing.
  - *Operative management:* ORIF with or without bone grafting.

■ **Os Supranaviculare**
- **Definition:** Accessory ossification center is located in the posterior superior aspect of the forefoot in 3.5% of patients.
- **Mechanism of Injury:** Shoes without arch support cause excessive pronation and irritate the bone. Tight shoelaces may also contribute.
- **Clinical Symptoms:** Swelling and pain over the medial foot at the location of the os.
- **Radiographs:** AP, lateral, or oblique films may show the os.
- **Treatment:** Ice and arch support. Steroid injection or surgical removal may be necessary.

■ **Spring Ligament Sprain**
- **Definition:** Medial midfoot sprain or injury to the calcaneal navicular ligament
- **Mechanism of Injury:** Often occurs from running on uneven ground or wearing lightweight shoes.
- **Clinical Symptoms:** Medial midfoot pain and aching.
- **Radiographs:** AP, oblique, and lateral views. Weight-bearing views may show widening between the tarsals and metatarsals.
- **Treatment:** Ice massage, NSAIDs, and posterior calf stretching. Strengthening of the foot intrinsic muscles. Proper footwear with medial heel wedge. Iontophoresis. May consider short term immobilization.

■ **Tarsal Coalition**
- **Definition:** Congenital fusion of the tarsal bones resulting in pain and a flat foot.
- **Mechanism of Injury:** Congenital. Often present with history of recurrent ankle sprains.
- **Clinical Symptoms:** Rigid, flat foot with pain below the ankle joint. Pain with activity.
- **Radiographs:** AP, lateral, and oblique foot films reveal a calcaneonavicular bar. CT scan is often helpful to show the extent of the fusion.
- **Treatment:** Orthotics with physical therapy for mild cases. Surgical resection of the bar and adhesions often required. Triple arthrodesis in severe cases.

■ **Tarsal Tunnel Syndrome (Tibial Nerve Entrapment)**
- **Definition:** The tarsal tunnel contents include the posterior tibial tendon, flexor digitorum longus tendon, flexor hallucis longus tendon, and the posterior tibial neurovascular bundle. The roof of the tunnel is made of the lacunate ligament going from the medial malleolus to the calcaneus. The floor is made of the tarsal bones and proximal metatarsals.
- **Mechanism of Injury:** Overuse from sporting activity causes nerve compression on the medial side of the foot.
- **Clinical Symptoms:** Medial posterior foot pain with burning and tingling of the toes. Worsened by standing or at night. Positive Tinel sign.
- **Radiographs:** Standard radiographs are usually not useful.
- **Treatment:** EMG may reveal prolonged nerve conduction of the medial plantar nerve. Medial arch support with medial wedge. Consider cortisone injection or cast immobilization. Surgical decompression for recalcitrant cases.

FOREFOOT AND TOES

■ **Fifth Metatarsal Injuries/Fracture**
- **Definition:** Injury at the base of the fifth metatarsal. Often seen with jumping sports or in athletes running on hard or uneven surfaces.
- **Mechanism of Injury:** Lateral inversion sprain of the ankle. Can present with one of three injuries:
  - Peroneus brevis strain
  - Avulsion fracture of the base of the fifth metatarsal
  - Jones fracture (transverse fracture through the fifth metatarsal diaphysis). May be stress fracture.
- **Clinical Symptoms:** Pain, swelling, and tenderness over the lateral foot. Antalgic gait.
- **Radiographs:** AP, lateral, and oblique views.
- **Treatment:**
  - *Peroneus brevis strain:* Eversion strapping, icing, NSAIDs.
  - *Avulsion fracture:* Immobilization with casting or walking boot for 1 to 3 weeks. Gradual return to activity as pain permits. Injury may heal with bony repair or fibrous tissue.

- * *Jones fracture:*
- * *Stress fracture:* May immobilize by casting or walking boot for 4 to 8 weeks.
  - * *Complete fracture:* Non-weight-bearing, SLC for 4 to 6 weeks. Surgical consideration with compression screw with or without bone grafting may also be an option.

▨ Metatarsalgia
- **Definition:** Vague term for metatarsal pain.
- **Mechanism of Injury:** Classified in two categories:
  1) *Primary:* Pain secondary to imbalance in weight distribution across metatarsals (hallux valgus, calluses, or shoe wear).
  2) *Secondary:* Joint imbalance by issues other than MTP joint dysfunction (metatarsal stress fracture, foot pronation, sesamoiditis, plantar fasciitis, Morton's foot).
- **Clinical Symptoms:** Pain or swelling across the metatarsals.
- **Radiographs:** Evaluate for causative disorder.
- **Treatment:** Per causative disorder.

▨ Metatarsal Stress Fracture
- **Definition:** Stress fracture developing in the metatarsal shaft. Most common in the 2nd or 5th metatarsal and in female athletes.
- **Mechanism of Injury:** Chronic repetitive stress such as in running or dancing or alteration in biomechanics secondary to blisters. Common in females and may be related to the FAT.
- **Clinical Symptoms:** Pain to palpation or percussion aggravated by plantarflexion or dorsiflexion.
- **Radiographs:** AP, lateral, or oblique views may be negative for first several weeks. Bone scan assists in the diagnosis and is positive within days. Also consider MRI.
- **Treatment:** Non-weight bearing or protected weight bearing until clinically healed. Correction of biomechanical factors.

▨ Morton Neuroma
- **Definition:** Nerve impingement of interdigital nerves at the site of the metatarsal head.
- **Mechanism of Injury:** Trauma and repetitive stress irritates the nerves. If it persists, an inflammatory tumor/neuroma may develop.
- **Clinical Symptoms:** Pain to palpation or burning sensation between metatarsal heads (usually between the 3rd and 4th metatarsal heads), which becomes worse with standing.
- **Radiographs:** Foot radiographs are not helpful.
- **Treatment:** Metatarsal pads to lift and separate metatarsal head, NSAIDs, or cortisone injection. Consideration for surgical excision if above treatment not successful.

▨ Osteochondrosis of Metatarsal Head ("Frieburg Disease")
- **Definition:** Injury to the vascular supply to the metatarsal head resulting in collapse. Commonly occurs in the second metatarsal head.

- **Mechanism of Injury:** Repetitive or acute stress to the metatarsal head.
- **Clinical Symptoms:** Localized pain and tenderness, worse with weight bearing.
- **Radiographs:** AP, lateral, and oblique radiographs show collapse of articular surface.
- **Treatment:** Metatarsal pad or bar to relieve stress, rigid foot plate insole, immobilization or surgical removal of metatarsal head in recalcitrant cases.

■ **Sesamoid Injuries**
- **Definition:** Inflammation and pain under the 1st metatarsal head in the location of the sesamoids located in the tendon of the flexor hallucis longus.
- **Mechanism of Injury:** Location of a cleat from a sport shoe (football, baseball, or soccer) under the sesamoids or dancing with bare feet. Hyperextension of the first MTP joint may present as acute fracture.
- **Clinical Symptoms:** Pain to palpation or with passive dorsiflexion of the great toe.
- **Radiographs:** AP, lateral, and oblique views of the great toe. If x-ray is negative and stress fracture is suspected, bone scan may be indicated. Sometimes there may be a normal variant of bipartite or tripartite sesamoids. MRI or bone scan.
- **Treatment:** Clinical suspicion suggests diagnosis. Taping, splinting, casting or orthotics along with ice, NSAIDs, and restricted weight-bearing.

■ **Turf Toe**
- **Definition:** Sprain of the joint capsule of the 1st MTP joint.
- **Mechanism of Injury:** May be caused by hyperdorsi- or hyperplantarflexion of the 1st MTP joint. Often related to sports participation on artificial turf.
- **Clinical Symptoms:** Pain reproduced by passive flexion or extension of the 1st MTP.
- **Radiographs:** Great toe radiographs are normal.
- **Treatment:** Taping toe to prevent flexion or extension of the 1st MTP, rigid foot plate insole, wear shoes with firm toe box, ice, NSAIDs, corticosteroid injection, iontophoresis.

PROCEDURES

■ **Morton's Neuroma Injection**
- **Indications:** Perineural fibrosis of interdigital nerve.
- **Patient Position:** Supine with towel under knee to create slight plantar flexion of foot.
- **Technique:** Approach nerve dorsally. Insert needle between metatarsal heads and advance through transverse tarsal ligament to a depth of approximately ½ inch.

■ **Plantar Fascia Injection**
- **Indications:** Recalcitrant Plantar fasciitis.
- **Patient Position:** Patient lies prone with foot supported in dorsiflexion.
- **Technique:** Identify medial calcaneal tubercle and needle inserted into medial side of soft part of sole just distal to heel pad.
- **Medicine/Needle::** 0.5-1 mLsteroid/1-2 mL anesthetic/25-27 gauge.

■ **Retrocalcaneal Bursae Injection**
- **Indications:** Retrocalcaneal bursitis.
- **Patient Position:** Patient lies prone with foot in slight dorsiflexion.
- **Technique:** Identify superior edge of calcaneus. Insert needle from lateral position just superior to calcaneus and anterior to Achilles tendon.
- **Medicine/Needle:** 0.5 mL steroid/1.5 mL anesthetic/23 gauge.

IV ■ MEDICAL INJURIES AND ILLNESSES

SPORTS CONCUSSION

NOTE: Universal agreement on definition and grading does not exist.
- **Definition:** Concussion or MTBI is a complex pathophysiologic process affecting the brain that is induced by direct or indirect biomechanical forces (2nd International Conference on Concussion in Sport, Prague, 2004). Common features include:
  - Rapid onset of usually short-lived neurologic impairment that typically resolves spontaneously.
  - Acute clinical symptoms that usually reflect a functional disturbance rather than structural injury.
  - A range of clinical symptoms that may or may not involve LOC.
  - Neuroimaging studies that are typically normal.

ACUTE CONCUSSION

- **Cognitive Features:** Confusion, amnesia, LOC, unaware of status of game.
- **Symptoms:** Headache, dizziness, feeling dazed, balance problems, nausea, visual problems, light sensitivity, ringing in ears, tiredness, confusion, disorientation, irritability or emotional changes, PTA.
- **Physical Signs:** LOC/impaired conscious state, gait unsteadiness, delayed response to questions, inability to follow directions, poor concentration, vomiting, vacant stare, slurred speech, significantly decreased playing ability, poor coordination or balance.
- **Most widely used guidelines:**
  - Summary and Agreement Statement of the International Conference on Concussion in Sport; Vienna, 2001 (1st); Prague, 2004 (2nd); Zurich, October 2008 (3rd).
  - Colorado Medical Society Sports Medicine Committee (1991).
  - American Academy of Neurology . (1997).
  - Cantu Evidence-Based Grading Scale (2001).

PRAGUE GUIDELINE SUMMARY (2004)

NOTE: Historical "grading" systems are not used.
- **Definition:** Sports concussion *is a complex pathophysiologic process affecting the brain induced by traumatic biomechanical forces.* Caused by direct blow to head face or neck, or elsewhere on the body with an "impulsive" force transmitted to the head
  - Typically results in rapid onset of short-lived impairment of neuro function that resolves spontaneously.
  - Largely reflect a functional disturbance rather than structural injury.

Colorado Medical Society Sports Medicine Committee (1991)

Grade	Features	Management	RTP
I	Confusion without amnesia No LOC	Remove from contest Examine immediately and at 5 min intervals for development of mental status abnormalities or post-concussive symptoms at rest or with exertion	May RTP if asymptomatic at rest and with exertion for at least 20 min 2nd grade I concussion in same contest: Disqualify athlete for that day 3rd grade I concussion: Terminate season
II	Confusion with amnesia No LOC	Remove from contest and disallow return that day Examine on site frequently for signs of evolving intracranial pathology CT or MRI if symptoms worsen or persist for longer than 1 week	May RTP after 1 full asymptomatic week at rest and with exertion 2nd grade II concussion: RTP after 1 month symptom free at rest and with exertion, consider termination of season 3rd grade II concussion: Terminate season
III	Any LOC	Transport athlete to nearest emergency department by ambulance with cervical spine precautions, if necessary	May return after 1 month if asymptomatic at rest and with exertion for at least 2 weeks 2nd grade III concussion: Terminate season, return to any contact sport seriously discouraged

AAN Grading System for Concussion (1997)

Grade	Features	Management	RTP
I	Transient confusion No LOC Concussion symptoms resolve in <15 min	Remove from contest Examine immediately and at 5-min intervals for development of mental status abnormalities or post-concussive symptoms at rest and with exertion	Return if clear within 15 min 2nd grade I in same contest: Disqualify athlete, return in 1 week if asymptomatic at rest and with exercise
II	Transient confusion No LOC Concussion symptoms last >15 min	Remove from contest and disallow return that day Examine on site frequently for signs of evolving intracranial pathology CT or MRI if symptoms worsen or persist for longer than 1 week	May return after 1 full asymptomatic week with exertion 2nd grade II concussion: RTP after 2 weeks symptom free at rest and with exertion
III	Any LOC, either brief (seconds) or prolonged (minutes)	Transport athletes to nearest emergency department by ambulance with cervical spine precautions, if necessary	Brief (seconds) grade III concussion: Withhold from play until asymptomatic for 2 weeks at rest and with exertion 2nd grade III concussion: Withhold from play for a minimum of 1 asymptomatic month

Cantu Data Driven Revised Concussion Guidelines (2001)

Grade	Features	Management	RTP
I	Transient confusion No LOC Concussion symptoms resolve in <30 min	Remove from contest Examine immediately and at 5-min intervals for development of mental status abnormalities or post-concussive symptoms at rest and with exertion	May RTP if asymptomatic for 1 week (rest and exertion) 2nd concussion: RTP in 2 weeks if asymptomatic at the time for 1 week (rest and exertion) 3rd concussion: Terminate season; may RTP next season if asymptomatic (rest and exertion)
II	Transient confusion LOC <1 min or PTA >30 min <24 h; other PCSS >30 min <7 days	Remove from contest and disallow return that day Examine on site frequently for signs of evolving intracranial pathology CT or MRI if symptoms worsen or persist for longer than 1 week	May RTP if asymptomatic for 1 week (rest and exertion) 2nd concussion: Minimum of 1 month; may RTP then if asymptomatic for 1 week (rest and exertion) 3rd concussion: Terminate season; may RTP next season if asymptomatic (rest and exertion)
III	LOC > 1 min or PTA > 24 h, PCSS > 7 days	Transport athletes to nearest emergency department by ambulance with cervical spine precautions, if necessary	Should not be allowed to play for at least 1 month. May RTP if asymptomatic for 1 week (rest and exertion) 2nd concussion: Terminate season; may RTP next season if asymptomatic

- Results in graded set of clinical syndromes with or without LOC.
- Resolution of symptoms typically follows a sequential course.
- Typically associated with grossly normal structural neuroimaging studies.
- LOC does not necessarily imply severity.
- Renewed interest in PTA as measure of severity.
- All concussions mandate evaluation by a medical doctor.

The 2004 Prague Guidelines classify concussions as either *simple* or *complex*.

■ Simple Concussion
- Most common.
- Injury resolves progressively without complication over 7 to 10 days.
- Limit playing or training time while symptomatic; no further intervention required.
- Formal NP screening not needed.
- Can be managed by PCP or ATC under medical supervision.
- Cornerstone of management is rest until all symptoms resolve and then graded program of exertion before return to sport.

■ Complex Concussion
- Prolonged cognitive impairment and persistent symptoms (including persistent symptoms recurrence with exertion), prolonged LOC (>1 minute).
- Includes athletes with multiple concussions received over time and/or repeated concussions with less impact force.
- Formal NP testing should be considered.
- Multidisciplinary management that includes specific expertise in concussion (i.e., sports neurologist, neurosurgeon, or neuropsychologist).

■ Prague Concussion Management
If any signs or symptoms of a concussion:
- Remove player from current game or practice.
- Do not leave patient unattended; monitor closely for initial few hours.
- Medical evaluation after injury.
- RTP must follow a medically supervised stepwise process.

■ Prague Stepwise RTP Protocol
- *Level 1*: No activity, complete rest, typically for a minimum of 24 hours. Once asymptomatic, proceed to level 2.
- *Level 2*: Light aerobic exercise (e.g., walking or stationary cycling, no resistance training).
- *Level 3*: Sport specific exercise (e.g., skating for hockey, running in soccer); progressive addition of resistance training at steps 3 and 4.
- *Level 4*: Non-contact training drills.
- *Level 5*: Full contact training drills after medical clearance.
- *Level 6*: Game play.

Note:
- Athlete may continue to proceed to next level if asymptomatic at current level.
- If any post-concussive symptoms occur, drop back to previous asymptomatic level and try to progress after 24 hours.
- Emphasize physical *and* cognitive rest
- With complex concussions: Rehabilitation is more prolonged and RTP more circumspect.

REMEMBER: Each concussion should be evaluated on an individual basis.

ACSM CONSENSUS STATEMENT (WWW.ACSM.ORG)

Return-to-Play (RTP) Decision:
- Individualized and not based on rigid timeline.
- Team physician ultimately responsible for RTP decision.

Same-Day RTP:
- Agreement that athlete should not RTP if significant or worsening signs or symptoms or ongoing RGA, PTA, or prolonged LOC.

Post-Game RTP:
- Determine if asymptomatic at rest before resuming any exertional activity.
- Progressive aerobic and resistance exercise challenge test before RTP.
- Factors affecting RTP:
- Severity of the injury
- Previous concussions
- Significant injury in response to a minor blow
- Age
- Sport
- Learning disabilities

OTHER RELATED ISSUES

■ Sideline Evaluation

Structured analysis and monitoring after injury should include:
- Assessing ABCs and potential for c-spine injury.
- Full neurologic exam including motor, cognitive functioning, memory testing.
- Standard orientation questions (time, place, and person) shown to be unreliable in the sporting situation compared to memory assessment.
- No athlete should RTP with any symptoms present at rest or with exertion.
- No RTP on same day if any LOC (even brief) or if symptoms still present after 15 to 20 minutes after injury.
- Frequent reevaluation and serial exams should be performed.
- "When in doubt, sit them out."

■ Concussion Prevention

- Concussions cannot be completely prevented.
- Helmet use decreases incidence of skull fracture and major trauma but does not decrease (and may increase) incidence of concussion.

- Improper use of head and helmet fit may increase risk of concussion.
- Rules to limit head trauma (e.g., no spearing, leading with head).
- Mouth guards may decrease severity.

■ During PPE
- Always obtain a detailed, specific history of prior concussion or symptoms of concussion after previous injury; athlete may not be aware of symptoms or may not have been "diagnosed" with a previous concussion.
- Baseline cognitive assessment at PPE for "high risk" sports (SCAT test vs. computerized NP testing).

■ Neuropsychologic (NP) Testing
- **Definition:** A cornerstone of diagnosis and management of sport concussion. NP testing may be limited or complex; e.g., a pen-and-paper test vs. computerized or formal testing with a neuropsychologist).
  - Post-injury testing can be compared to pre-season baseline test scores if available.
  - Test after becoming asymptomatic and RTP.
  - Consider if PCSS present for >7 days or sooner as indicated.
  - Adopted by the NHL, NFL, MLB, NASCAR, and some NBA and collegiate teams.

■ Neuroimaging
Imaging is not essential for simple concussive injury (results are usually normal) but should be used when suspicious of intracerebral structural lesions. Consider imaging if:
  - Prolonged post-concussive symptoms
  - Focal neurological deficit or worsening symptoms
Promising imaging technologies (PET, SPECT, and fMRI) are in the early stages of research and development.

■ Post-concussive Syndrome
- **Definition:** Persistent concussion symptoms lasting weeks or months following a head injury.
- **Diagnosis:** Symptoms may include headache, blurred vision, depression, fatigue, sleep disturbance, poor memory, decreased appetite, anxiety.
  - Neurologic exam is usually normal
  - Neuropsychologic testing, neuroimaging, and treatment may be indicated.
- **Treatment:** Symptom-dependent and can include analgesics, SSRIs.
Most athletes will have complete resolution of symptoms in 3 to 6 months.

■ Second Impact Syndrome
Controversial topic.
- **Definition:** Minor head injury is followed (before symptoms resolve) by a second concussive injury with subsequent rapid neurologic deterioration and death within hours of the second head injury. Second injury may be minor. Most susceptible in adolescents.
- **Diagnosis:** Athlete may have symptoms similar to a mild concussion for seconds to minutes.

- Catastrophic brain injury thought to be secondary to loss of cerebral autoregulation with cerebral edema and subsequent brainstem herniation within seconds to minutes.
- Deterioration occurs more rapidly than may be seen with an epidural hematoma.
- **Treatment:** Transport to medical facility for treatment: Immediate intubation, hyperventilation, and osmotic diuretic.

OTHER HEAD INJURIES

■ Epidural Hematoma
- **Definition:** Most commonly results from a tear of the middle meningeal artery. Associated with a skull fracture 80% of the time.
- **Diagnosis:** Epidural hematoma is classically associated with a lucid interval, i.e., initial LOC followed by a period of full use of faculties followed by rapid neurologic deterioration.
- **Treatment:** Immediate transfer to an appropriate facility is required for neurosurgical consultation.

■ Skull Fractures
- **Definition:** Skull fractures may be open or closed. Always be aware of possible intracranial hemorrhage.
- **Diagnosis:** An obvious bony step-off may be palpated along with signs of hemotympanum, battle's sign (ecchymosis behind the ear), and raccoon eyes (ecchymosis under the eyes). Also examine for CSF leakage from nares.
- **Treatment:** Hairline fracture with no depression and no CSF leaks may be managed by sports medicine doctor. Any depressed fracture or CSF leak can cause neurologic problems or increased risk of infection and require neurosurgical consult.

■ Subarachnoid Hemorrhage
- **Definition:** Bleeding located between the arachnoid and the pia mater. Usually results from trauma but can be from non-traumatic etiologies such as aneurysms.
- **Diagnosis:** Symptoms include headache, possible LOC, and other severe neurologic deficits that can occur rapidly. Non-traumatic forms sometimes present with a "thunderclap" headache or "worse headache of my life." Head CT should be performed; if negative, lumbar puncture should be considered.
- **Treatment:** Requires hospitalization and imaging.

■ Subdural Hematoma
- **Definition:** More common than an epidural hematoma. This injury results from a disruption of bridging venous blood vessels.

- **Diagnosis:** Can be associated with LOC and focal neurologic deficits. Can present hours to days after head trauma due to slow venous bleed.
- **Treatment:** Immediate transfer to an appropriate facility for neurosurgical consultation.

FACIAL INJURIES

■ Epistaxis
- **Definition:** Roughly 90% of all nose bleeds are anterior. Most common site for bleeding is Kiesselbach plexus.
- **Diagnosis:** Bleeding from one or both nares.
- **Treatment:** Initially, compression of the nose while leaning head forward. If bleeding stops, may RTP. If bleeding persists, may use nasal sprays with neo-synephrine or lidocaine with epinephrine, as both will cause vasoconstriction. Silver nitrate may be used if bleed can be located. Nasal packing with nasal tampon should be left in place for 3 to 5 days.

■ Lip Laceration
- **Definition:** Occurs frequently in sporting events. Increased vascularity and the need for cosmetic results require a careful assessment.
- **Diagnosis:** Clinical based on examination. Need to include exam of lips and oral mucosa.
- **Treatment:** Most injuries to the lip and oral mucosa heal very well without any sutures. If the injury involves the vermillion border, then special care must be taken to ensure that the border will heal well approximated. Suture the vermillion border first if required. A field block around the lips is recommended to ensure no distortion of anatomic landmarks.

■ Mandibular Fractures
- **Definition:** Relatively common fractures involved with high speed trauma.
- **Diagnosis:** Increased motion of jaw, malocclusion, paresthesia of lower lip. X-rays of jaw for diagnosis. CT scan, if x-rays negative but still suspicious.
- **Treatment:** On-site treatment requires immobilization of possible fracture. This can be achieved using Ace-wrap. Transport and referral to ENT required. Usually ORIF.

■ Maxillary Fractures
- **Definition:** Involve upper jaw. These fractures are the result of direct blow to middle portion of face.
- **Diagnosis:** Increased mobility of maxilla and midface, biting malocclusion and ecchymosis. Epistaxis and nasal deformity also possible. CT scan is the gold standard, but x-ray including Waters view may be helpful.
- **Treatment:** Classification is Le Fort I, II, and III. Usually requires surgery, possibly secondary reconstruction.

■ **Nasal Fracture**
- **Definition:** Most common sports-related facial fracture. Look for acute pain, epistaxis, and ecchymosis.
- **Diagnosis:** Examination may show nasal deformity. Use nasal speculum to exam the septum for septal hematoma.
- **Treatment:** Consists of reduction if done immediately or referral to ENT within 5 to 7 days. Athletes should not RTP on same day as injury. Workouts restricted if nasal packing present. Participation in contact sports may need to be restricted unless the fracture can be protected by a shield.

■ **Septal Hematoma**
- **Definition:** A rare, possible complication of a nasal fracture or reducing the fracture. Is considered an emergency as it can cause long-term saddle nose defect due to pressure necrosis. Monitor for infection.
- **Diagnosis:** Patient will have pain with nasal obstruction. May see bluish discoloration and bulging on the medial surface of the septum.
- **Treatment:** Obtain ENT consultation. Immediate drainage after anesthesia using an 18- to 20-gauge needle required. Nasal packing to prevent recurrence and prophylactic antibiotics are recommended.

ENT

■ **Auricular Hematoma**
- **Definition:** Associated with athletes in boxing, wrestling and rugby. Can be caused by direct trauma and increased friction in activity.
- **Diagnosis:** Ear initially becomes swollen and painful and develops a fluctuant or tense hematoma.
- **Treatment:** Drainage, pressure dressing for 7 to 10 days to prevent recurrence, and prophylactic antibiotics. No RTP until after pressure dressing is removed.

■ **Avulsed Tooth**
- **Definition:** Tooth that has been ripped completely out of socket.
- **Diagnosis:** Confirmed by physical examination. The periodontal ligaments are torn but the cells from the periodontal ligament must be protected.
- **Treatment:** Re-implantation within 30 minutes increases survival rate of the tooth to 90%. If re-implantation cannot be achieved, then transport to dentist in saliva, milk, or other proper medium.

■ **Tooth Fracture**
- **Definition:** Fracture of the enamel and/or dentin of the tooth.
- **Diagnosis:** Visualization of enamel (which is white), dentin (mostly yellow) and pulp (which is red) is necessary. Also examine for possible maxillary or mandibular injury.
- **Treatment:** Tooth fractures are characterized based on location; root, crown, and chipped tooth. Most serious is injury to pulp characterized by significant sensitivity, including to air. Pulp and dentin involvement

require immediate treatment and no RTP. Injury to enamel can RTP but need follow up within 24 to 48 hours.

■ **Tympanic Membrane Rupture**
- **Definition:** Athlete has history of some form of barotrauma. Can result in partial or total loss of hearing.
- **Diagnosis:** Easily diagnosed with otoscope. Be sure to document location of the rupture along with relative size.
- **Treatment:** 90% of ruptures heal within 8 weeks. Some recommend oral antibiotics if injury was in seawater. Others propose better healing with use of decongestants. If no healing occurs within 8 to 12 weeks, then ENT referral is needed for possible tympanoplasty.

EYE INJURIES

■ **Corneal Abrasion**
- **Definition:** History of trauma associated with significant pain, photophobia, and a sense of a foreign body in the eye.
- **Diagnosis:** After using anesthetic drops, fluorescein stain on the cornea will help visualize the abrasion. A Wood lamp or slit lamp can be used to visualize the staining. Always evert the eyelid to rule out an occult foreign body.
- **Treatment:** If an abrasion is seen, antibiotic drops are used as treatment at home. Mydriatic drops and anesthetic may only be used in the clinic. Follow up in 24 to 48 hours to ensure healing. Patching is not usually indicated. Pain control with oral narcotics may be indicated.

■ **Foreign Body in the Eye**
- **Definition:** A careful history regarding the nature of the injury and type of foreign body is important.
- **Diagnosis:** Always evert the eyelid for evaluation. Check for visual acuity. Fluorescein stain may also be indicated..
- **Treatment:** A sterile cotton-tipped applicator moistened with saline may be used to remove the foreign body. One may also use the tip of an 18- to 22-gauge needle. Ophthalmology referral may be necessary if foreign body removal involves the visual axis.

■ **Hyphema**
- **Definition:** Common ocular injury resulting in collection of blood in the anterior chamber of the eye. Associated with severe ocular trauma; full examination is required.
- **Diagnosis:** Blood in the anterior chamber can be easily visualized upon examination. Need to check intra-ocular pressure.
- **Treatment:** Ophthalmologic management necessary due to possible complications of glaucoma. Strict bed rest recommended. Atropine can be used for pain. Risk of recurrent bleed is highest days 3 to 5.

- ■ **Orbital Wall Fracture**
  - **Definition:** Results from significant trauma to the eye. Usually located in the floor of the orbit. Patient will complain of significant pain along with swelling and superior gaze diplopia.
  - **Diagnosis:** A full eye examination, focusing on extra-ocular motion, facial numbness and bony crepitus.
  - **Treatment:** Eye shielding along with immediate antibiotics and transport are needed. CT scan is the gold standard for diagnosis, but a Waters view may be used. Immediate surgical intervention needed with loss of extra-ocular movement or large fracture.

- ■ **Retinal Detachment**
  - **Definition:** Due to transferred force from impact, a tear in the retina takes place. Symptoms start as blind spot at edge of visual field. One can see "flashing lights," and then "floaters."
  - **Diagnosis:** Visual fields examination must be done for any possible defects. A indirect fundoscopic exam with a dilated eye by an ophthalmologist is indicated.
  - **Treatment:** Referral to ophthalmologist is required for appropriate dilation and visualization of the defect. Laser treatment is used to stop any further tearing of the retina.

- ■ **Ruptured Globe**
  - **Definition:** Results from direct significant trauma to the globe of the eye. These can present with orbital fractures.
  - **Diagnosis:** Visual inspection of the globe reveals an area of leaking fluid of light or dark color. Visual acuity along with palpation or orbital rims required.
  - **Treatment:** Referral to ophthalmologist is required. Place an eye shield over injured eye and transport to nearest appropriate medical facility.

CARDIAC INJURIES

CARDIOLOGY AND SPORTS MEDICINE

Treating cardiac abnormalities is a complex task for the sports medicine practitioner. Consultation with a sports cardiologist may be necessary. Familiarity with the *36th Bethesda Conference Guidelines: Eligibility Recommendations for Competitive Athletes with Cardiovascular Abnormalities* (2005) is necessary to provide pertinent information to the individual with an identified cardiovascular abnormality. The expert panel ascertains the abnormalities and severity that will place competitive athletes at risk for SCD.

The Bethesda Conference Guidelines are revised periodically. The reasons for the current revisions are:

1) Substantial advances in the diagnosis and management of a variety of genetic and acquired cardiovascular diseases.
2) Impact of ethical and legal issues on medical decision making.

3) SCD continues to be a highly visible, compelling, and emotional event with significant liability considerations.

SUDDEN CARDIAC DEATH DEMOGRAPHICS

- Occurs in both genders but men > women (9:1)
- Occurs in all races
- Occurs in variety of ages
- Occurs in broad spectrum of sports (particularly basketball and football in the United States and soccer in Europe)

Although 10 to 15 million athletes participate in organized sports in the United States, the number of athletes who die of cardiovascular or related causes is less than 300/year.

36TH BETHESDA CONFERENCE DESIGN AND FORMAT

- *Task Force 1*: Pre-participation Screening
- *Task Force 2*: Congenital Heart Disease
- *Task Force 3*: Valvular Heart Disease
- *Task Force 4*: HCM and Other Cardiomyopthies, MVP, Myocarditis, and Marfan Syndrome
- *Task Force 5*: Systemic Hypertension
- *Task Force 6*: Coronary Artery Disease
- *Task Force 7*: Arrhythmias
- *Task Force 8*: Classification of Sports
- *Task Force 9*: Drugs and Performance-Enhancing Substances
- *Task Force 10*: Automated External Defibrillators
- *Task Force 11*: Commotio Cordis
- *Task Force 12*: Legal Aspects of the 36th Bethesda Conference Recommendations

TASK FORCE 1: PRE-PARTICIPATION SCREENING AND DIAGNOSIS OF CARDIOVASCULAR DISEASE

■ **Objectives of PPE Screening:**
- Recognition of "silent" CV abnormalities
- Evaluation of an heart murmur
- Cardiac symptoms (exertional chest pain, dyspnea, syncope)
- Family history

AMERICAN HEART ASSOCIATION RECOMMENDATIONS OF CARDIAC PRE-PARTICIPATION

■ **Athletic Screening:**
- Family history
  - Premature SCD
  - Heart disease in surviving relatives <50 years old
- Personal history
  - Heart murmur
  - Systemic hypertension

- Fatigue
- Syncope/near-syncope
- Excessive/unexplained exertional dyspnea
- Exertional chest pain
- Physical examination
  - Heart murmur (supine/standing)
  - Femoral arterial pulses (to exclude coarctation of aorta)
  - Stigmata of Marfan syndrome
  - Brachial BP measurement (sitting)

TASK FORCE 2: CONGENITAL HEART DISEASE
- Atrial septal defect (ASD)
- Ventricular septal defect (VSD)
- Patent ductus arteriosis (PDA)
- Pulmonary valve stenosis (PS)
- Aortic valve stenosis (AS)
- Coarctation of the aorta
- Elevated pulmonary resistance with congenital heart disease
- Tetrology of Fallot
- Cyanotic congenital cardiac disease
- Transposition of the great arteries (TGA)
- Congenitally connected transposition of the great arteries (CCTGA)
- Ebstein's anomaly
- Congenital coronary artery anomalies (CCAA)

TASK FORCE 3: VALVULAR HEART DISEASE
- Mitral stenosis
- Mitral regurgitation
- Aortic stenosis
- Aortic regurgitation
- Tricuspic regurgitation
- Multivalvular disease
- Valve repair or replacement

TASK FORCE 4: HCM AND OTHER CARDIOMYOPATHIES, MITRAL VALVE PROLAPSE, MYOCARDITIS, AND MARFAN SYNDROME
- Hypertrophic cardiomyopathy
- Mitral valve prolapse (MVP)
- Myocarditis
- Marfan syndrome
- Ehlers-Danlos syndrome
- Arrhythmogenic right ventricular cardiomyopathy (AVRC)
- Pericarditis
- Anomalous coronary artery. Types of anomalies:
  - Single coronary artery
  - Coronary artery hypoplasia

- Origin of coronary from pulmonary artery
- Anomalous coronary artery

TASK FORCE 5: SYSTEMIC HYPERTENSION

- Most common CV condition in competitive athletes
- In patients >18 years old, HTN = 140/90
- HTN by itself has not been implicated as a cause of SCD
- BP obtained in the seated position. Sit quietly for 5 minutes with back supported and feet on floor with arm at level of the heart.
- No caffeine ~ 1 hour
- No smoking ~ 30 minutes
- Cuff size: Bladder should cover 80% of length of arm
- Take at least two readings. If readings vary by >55 mm Hg, take additional readings.
- Take pressure in both arms and use higher pressure.

TASK FORCE 6: CORONARY ARTERY DISEASE

- Atherosclerotic coronary artery disease
- Coronary artery vasospasm
- CAD in cardiac transplant recipients

TASK FORCE 7: TYPES OF ARRHYTHMIAS

- Disturbances of sinus node function
- Premature atrial complexes
- Atrial flutter (in absence of WPW)
- Atrial fibrillation (in absence of WPW)
- AV junctional escape beats/rhythm
- Premature AV junctional complexes
- Non-paroxysmal AV junctional tachycardia
- Supraventricular tachycardia
- Ventricular pre-excitation
- Premature ventricular complexes
- Ventricular tachycardia (VT)
- First-degree AV block
- Type 1 second-degree (Wenckebach) AV block
- Type 2 second-degree (Mobitz) AV block
- Congenital complete heart block
- Acquired complete heart block
- Complete right bundle-branch block
- Complete left bundle-branch block
- Inherited arrhythmia syndromes
- Long QT syndrome
- Short QT syndrome
- Catecholaminergic polymorphic ventricular tachycardia (CPVT)
- Brugada syndrome (BrS)

TASK FORCE 8: CLASSIFICATION OF SPORTS

Refer to http://www.acc.org/qualityandscience/clinical/bethesda/beth36/index.pdf for specific information.

TASK FORCE 9: DRUGS AND PERFORMANCE-ENHANCING SUBSTANCES

Refer to http://www.acc.org/qualityandscience/clinical/bethesda/beth36/index.pdf for specific information.

TASK FORCE 10: AUTOMATED EXTERNAL DEFIBRILLATORS (AEDS)

- AEDs at sites of training and competition
- AEDs should be available at education facilities that have competitive athletic programs
- Response time <5 minutes
- Initial response for cardiac arrest
- Call 911
- Initiate CPR
- Deploy the AED

TASK FORCE 11: COMMOTIO CORDIS

Refer to http://www.acc.org/qualityandscience/clinical/bethesda/beth36/index.pdf for specific information.

TASK FORCE 12: LEGAL ASPECTS OF THE 36TH BETHESDA CONFERENCE GUIDELINES

Refer to http://www.acc.org/qualityandscience/clinical/bethesda/beth36/index.pdf for specific information.

KEY CARDIAC CONDITIONS IN SPORTS MEDICINE

■ **Sudden Death in Exercise**
- **Definition:** Rare, nontraumatic death during or within 1 hour following participation in athletics that is not a result of bodily injury.
  - Male:female (9:1)
  - College athletes:high school athletes (2:1)
  - "Younger athlete" (age <35 years): Most often associated with congenital CV structural anomalies.
  - "Older athlete" (age >35 years): Over 75% from acquired atherosclerotic CAD

■ **Hypertrophic Cardiomyopathy**
- **Definition:** A cardiovascular condition that is the most common etiology of SCD for those <35 years. Accounts for 1/3 of cardiac deaths in the United States and is found in 0.2% of the general population. Defined as asymmetric hypertrophy associated with a non-dilated LV and a maximal LV end-diastolic wall thickness of 15 mm or more in the adult athlete.

Causes of SCD during Exercise in Athletes

Conditions causing myocardial ischemia
Atherosclerotic CAD
Coronary artery spasm
Coronary artery dissection
Anomalous coronary arteries
Hypoplastic coronary arteries

Structural abnormalities
HCM
Mitral valve prolapse
Aortic stenosis
Valvular heart disease
Idopathic concentric LVH
Marfan syndrome – aortic rupture
RV dysplasis

Arrhythmias
WPW
Long QT syndrome
Ventricular arrhythmias
Genetic conductive abnormalities
Arrhythmogenic RV cardiomyopathy*

Miscellaneous
Myocarditis
Sickle cell trait
Commotio cordis
Substance abuse – cocaine or steroids
Sarcoidosis

*More commonly recognized in European studies

- **Diagnosis:** Prodromal symptoms of presyncope or syncope with or without exertion may be present. Systolic murmur is often present; increases with Valsalva maneuver. Athletes must be screened during PPE for any family history of sudden death, prodromal symptoms, and murmurs.
- **Tests:** ECHO is generally diagnostic; abnormal ECG findings can be non-specific.
- **Treatment:** Cardiology consult; beta blockers; surgical; septal artery ethanol ablation; implanted defibrillators

HCM versus Athlete's Heart

HCM		Athlete's Heart
+	Unusual patterns of LVH	-
+	LV cavity < 45 mm*	-
-	LV cavity > 55 mm*	+
+	Marked LA enlargement	-
+	Abnormal ECG patterns	-
+	Abnormal LV filling	-
+	Female gender	-
-	↓thickness with deconditioning	+
+	Family history of HCM	-
-	Max. VO_2 > 45 mL/kg/min	+

* "Gray zone" of LV wall thickness (13 to 15 mm).

- **RTP:** Athletes with confirmed cases should not be given clearance to play. Low-intensity sports are an option for some.
- ■ **Congenital Coronary Artery Abnormalities (CCAA)**
  - **Definition:** Cardiac vascular anomalies responsible for up to 20% of causes of sudden death in young athletes—second after HCM. Prevalence in 0.2% to 1% of the general population. Mechanism of death is myocardial ischemia.
  - **Types:**
    - Anomalous origin of the left main coronary from the right sinus of Valsalva (most common)
    - Single coronary artery
    - Origin of the coronary artery from pulmonary artery
    - Coronary artery hypoplasia
  - **Diagnosis:** Symptoms include fatigue, exertional chest pain, or exercise-induced syncope; found in < 30% of patients. ECG changes rarely detected; anomalies detected by ECHO or angiogram.
  - **Treatment:** Dependant on age and symptoms, surgical repair of malformation.
- ■ **Athletic Heart Syndrome (AHS)**
  - **Definition:** Benign cardiac structural and physiologic adaptive changes to athletic training. May be hard to distinguish from possible underlying pathologic condition.

- *Endurance-trained athletes*: Increased left ventricular wall thickness, eccentric hypertrophy, decreased resting HR from improved CO.
- *Strength-trained athlete*: Concentric hypertrophy, increased wall thickness without significant change in end-diastolic diameter.
- **Diagnosis:**
  - HR: 40 to 60 BPM secondary to enhanced vagal tone and decreased sympathetic tone. -
  - Physiologic S2 split during inspiration.
  - S3 may be noted in endurance-trained athletes (increased rate of LV filling associated with dilatation).
  - S4 may be noted in strength-trained athletes secondary to concentric hypertrophy. This warrants clinical evaluation; 30% to 50% may have functional murmurs.
  - 40% have abnormal ECGs.
- **Treatment:** No treatment needed though detraining for 2 to 3 months can result in reversal of these changes.

Common ECG Findings in AHS

Sinus bradycardia	Incomplete RBBB
RVH voltage criteria	Tall, peaked, and inverted T waves
Notched P waves	LVH by voltage criteria
QTc interval at upper limit	Wenckebach AV block
Sinus arrhythmia	Repolarization changes

Features of AHS versus Cardiomyopathy

Feature	AHS	Cardiomyopathy
LVH	<13 mm	>15 mm
LV end-diastolic diameter	<60 mm	>70 mm
Diastolic function	Normal (E:A ratio >1)	Abnormal (E:A ratio <1)
Septal hypertrophy	Symmetric	Asymmetric (in HCM)
Family history	None	May be present
BP response to exercise	Normal	Normal or reduced systolic response
Deconditioning	LV hypertrophy regression	No LV hypertrophy regression

■ **Hypertension (HTN) in Athletes**
- **Definition:** BP >140/90 and the most common CV condition in competitive athletes.
- **Diagnosis:** Workup and treatment are no different than with the non-athlete.

NOTE: Use care not to over diagnose in young athletes and use proper cuff size with 3 different measures on 3 different days.

- **Treatment:** Medication, lifestyle and dietary changes.
- **RTP:** Mild to moderate HTN with no target organ damage or heart disease should not limit eligibility for participation. They should be followed closely and receive treatment. Athletes with severe HTN should be treated and readings should reach an appropriate level before clearance is given.

■ **Mitral Valve Prolapse (MVP)**
- **Definition:** Most common heart valve abnormality affecting 5% to 10% of the population. Valve leaflets prolapse into the atrium allowing leakage (regurgitation). Asymptomatic in most people.
- **Diagnosis:** Murmur. Asymptomatic in most people. Symptoms may include fatigue, palpitations, chest pain, anxiety, headaches.
- **Sports Participation:** MVP precludes participation only if one of the following is present (see 36th Bethesda Guidelines for Athletic Participation):
  - History of arrhythmia with syncope
  - Family history of sudden death that is MVP related
  - History of embolic event
  - Arrhythmia exacerbated by exercise
  - Moderate to severe mitral regurgitation

Considerations need to be made on an individual basis; consider low-intensity sport if any of the above applies.

■ **Myocarditis**
- **Definition:** Inflammation of the myocardium.
  - Cause of 20% of SCD secondary to ventricular arrhythmia.
  - Generally secondary to viral or bacterial infection (coxsackie B in 50% of cases); also from immune-mediated disease (Kawasaki or acute rheumatic fever), collagen vascular disease. Chronic cocaine use linked with histologic features of myocarditis.
  - Exercise during coxsackie infection increases risk of myocarditis in animal studies.
  - Few, if any, prodromal signs or symptoms but may include:
  - Recent viral infection.

NOTE: Consider withholding athletes with viral infection from exercise while any systemic symptoms are present (fever, myalgias, etc.)
  - Fever, myalgias
  - Chest pain
  - Shortness of breath
  - Exercise intolerance

- CHF, dyspnea, cough, and orthopnea
- **Diagnosis:** Symptoms may include:
  - Fever
  - Palpitations (due to arrhythmias)
  - Pericarditis
  - S3 gallop, soft apical murmur, distended neck veins, peripheral edema
  - Labs: Elevated CRP, ESR; elevated markers of myocardial damage: CK, troponin
  - ECG: T-wave inversions, saddle-shaped ST-segment elevations
  - ECHO: Reveals enlargement of the heart chambers and impaired LV function
- **Treatment:** Rest, diuretics, inotropes, digoxin, afterload reduction, steroids, gamma globulin. Withdraw from competitive activity for up to 6 months with RTP only after cardiology consult.

■ Commotio Cordis

- **Definition:** Another cause of sudden death in athletes as a result of a blunt, innocent-appearing, anterior chest wall trauma leading to ventricular fibrillation and usually instantaneous cardiac arrest. Primarily an "electric event" with autopsy absent of any significant cardiac or thoracic injury.
  - Contusio cordis is a "myocardial contusion" or tissue damage due to high impact blows that also result in injury to the overlying structures of the chest and thorax.
- **Diagnosis:**
  - Second leading cause of death in youth athletics; mean age 14 years old.
  - Higher risk because of pliability of chest wall in youth.
  - Timely blow (from ball, puck, helmet, punch, etc.) during a vulnerable window before the T-wave peak, with velocity, location, and hardness of impact crucial variables.
  - Most commonly seen in baseball but can be seen in any sport (high incidence in lacrosse, ice hockey, softball, soccer, karate, football).
- **Treatment:** Successful resuscitation can be achieved only with early defibrillation. Overall survival rate is poor. Survivors should undergo a thorough cardiac evaluation .
- **Prevention:** Incidence may be decreased using some types of protective equipment (commercially available chest protectors ineffective; "safety" baseballs up to age 13 reduce risk). Emphasis should be on more widespread availability of automated external defibrillators (AEDs).
- **RTP:** Is left to clinical judgment.

■ Marfan Syndrome

- **Definition:** Genetic disorder of connective tissue with a predisposition to CV abnormalities, specifically affecting the heart valves and aorta.
  - Up to 90% of the mortality attributed to Marfan syndrome is related to CV complications; i.e., mitral valve regurgitation or occult progressive

dilation of the aorta and subsequent aortic regurgitation, dissection, or rupture.

- **Diagnosis:** Screen males >6 feet and women >5 feet 10 inches tall or suspicious body habitus. Murmur from MV prolapse and/or aortic regurgitation (diastolic murmur). *Need two of these four major features:*
  1) Family history
  2) CV abnormality (murmur or mid-systolic click, aortic aneurysm, MVP, congestive heart failure symptoms)
  3) Musculoskeletal abnormality (arm span > height, kyphoscoliosis, anterior thoracic deformity, arched palate)
  4) Ocular abnormalities (myopia, ectopic lens)
- **Tests:** Consider ECHO and slit lamp exam if suspicious; genetic and cardiology consult. Goal of treatment is to slow progression of aortic dilation and damage to valves; beta blockers, surgery. May have to restrict from athletics.

■ When to Consider ECHO Evaluation

Not recommended at this time for routine screening. Conditions in which an ECHO may be useful in evaluating an athlete:

- HCM
- Unexplained heart murmur; increased with squat-to-stand test
- Unexplained abnormal ECG
- Pericarditis
- Myocarditis
- Suspected congenital heart disease
- Anomalies of the coronary arteries
- Suspected valvular disease
- Arrhythmias

PULMONARY

■ Asthma

- **Definition:** Caused by intermittent narrowing of the airways secondary to endobronchial inflammation and bronchial smooth muscle hyperactivity/constriction.
- **Diagnosis:** Symptoms include cough, wheezing, shortness of breath, chest tightness, chest pain, and difficulty breathing. Any or all of these symptoms may be present. Diagnosis consists of symptoms as listed and demonstrating reversible airway obstruction. This may be done through peak flow measurements and/or spirometry. IOC requires lab testing to support diagnosis. Eucapneic voluntary hyperventilation more sensitive than methocholine challenge testing.
- **Treatment:**
  - Inhaled bronchodilators
  - Inhaled steroids
  - Combination agents (i.e., fluticasone and salmeterol)

stic Fibrosis (CF)

- **Definition:** An autosomal recessive disorder characterized by thick bronchial mucus production.
- **Diagnosis:** It causes progressive airway obstruction, inflammation, infections with eventual pulmonary fibrosis. Many CF patients will have a productive cough with exercise. This can be beneficial in clearing mucus and opening the bronchial airways. It is not contagious and not a hazard to teammates, coaches, etc.
- **Treatment:** Special attention should be made to hydration/electrolytes as they may have difficulty with salt/water regulation. More severe CF patients may require supplemental O_2. However, people with CF should still be encouraged to participate in athletics/exercise programs with proper knowledge and understanding of the disease.

■ Exercise-Induced Asthma (EIA)

- **Definition:** People with EIA typically show asthma symptoms during or after exercise or physical exertion.
- **Diagnosis:** Symptoms and airflow obstruction tend to be transient in nature, lasting 30 to 60 minutes following exercise completion with resolution shortly thereafter. Symptoms at rest should raise suspicion of chronic asthma. Other factors that may influence severity of symptoms include cold temperature, dry climates, tobacco smoke, and other environmental allergens.
- **Tests:**
  - *Empiric Treatment*: Therapeutic trial with beta-agonist or cromolyn sodium prior to exercise with symptomatic improvement or lack of symptoms after or during exertion is suggestive of EIA.
  - *Pulmonary Function Tests (PFTs)*: Evaluate peak expiratory flow (PEF), forced expiratory volumes in 1 second (FEV1)/ forced vital capacity (FVC) and forced expiratory flow 25-75% (FEF 25-75). FEV1 typically normal in pre-exercise individuals and <80% in chronic asthmatics. Good for baseline but not ideal for EIA diagnosis as a stand alone test.
  - *Exercise Challenge*: Exercise to achieve 80% to 90% of maximal heart rate for 5 to 10 minutes (should be sport specific). Measure FEV1, FVC, and FEF 25-75 immediately post exercise and at 3 to 5 minute intervals for 20 to 30 minutes. ↓FEV1 ≥15% is diagnostic.
  - *Methacholine Challenge*: Nebulized methacholine is administered which lowers FEV1 and pulmonary function. A higher dose is needed for non-asthmatics. Can be used when standard PFTs/exercise challenge results are equivocal.
  - *Eucapnic Voluntary Hyperventilation*: Approved by IOC. Most sensitive test in elite athletes. Dry gas (O_2, N, and CO_2) is inhaled at a rate of 85% maximum voluntary ventilation for 6 minutes. ↓ FEV1 ≥20% is diagnostic.
- **Treatment:** Inhaled short-acting beta agonists (albuterol/terbutaline) remain the first line treatment. 1 to 2 puffs 15 to 30 minutes prior to

exercise with 2 to 4 hour duration. Mast cell stabilizers (cromolyn/nedocromil) alone or in conjunction with beta agonists may also be beneficial. Be aware of banned substances or regulations depending on level of competition. Switching sports to a less intense/exertional activity may give some relief of symptoms. The athlete may take advantage of the refractory period by performing warm-up activities, short sprints, or prolonged submaximal exercise, 45 to 60 minutes prior to competition. In cold air climates the athlete may use scarf/mask to limit cold air exposure. Avoid exposure to predetermined triggers/allergens.

Hyperventilation Syndrome

- **Definition:** Most common in anxiety/panic/stressful situations causing an increase in respiratory rate and subsequent hyperventilation. Prolonged hyperventilation causes a decreased PCO_2 and an increase in arterial pH.
- **Diagnosis:** The patient may complain of dyspnea, faintness, confusion, extremity numbness, and/or paresthesias. Aside from tachypnea there are no specific physical exam findings. Lab tests are usually not helpful; however, PFTs, if readily available, may provide assistance.
- **Treatment:** Treatment consists of reassuring the patient and advising the patient to breathe slowly or breathe into a bag to raise alveolar CO_2.

Pneumothorax

- **Definition:** Typically seen in contact sports such as hockey, football, and lacrosse. Described as air present in the pleural space between the lung and chest wall. May be spontaneous, result from congenital bleb rupture or direct trauma. Spontaneous pneumothorax is more common among young, thin males.
- **Diagnosis:** Typically present with acute dyspnea with mild shortness of breath. More severe cases may have more severe dyspnea, acute pleuritic chest pain, cough, and severe shortness of breath. Findings on exam may include absent breath sounds on affected side, wheezing, or overall poor air exchange. A tension pneumothorax may also cause tracheal deviation, hypotension, unilateral loss of breath sounds, distended neck veins, and possible cyanosis. Diagnosis is usually made through clinical suspicion based on history and classic exam findings and confirmed with CXR (PA and lateral decubitus with suspected side uppermost).
- **Treatment:** Treatment varies depending on size. Findings ≤20% may be treated with careful observation, supplemental O_2, and close follow-up including x-rays. ≥20% typically requires hospitalization and chest tube placement. Tension pneumothorax should be immediately treated with needle decompression. Return to non-contact activity is about 3 to 6 weeks following resolution, with special consideration with flying and scuba diving.

Pulmonary Contusion

- **Definition:** Generally results from a blunt injury to the chest wall with subsequent injury to lung parenchyma. This leads to edema and blood collection in the alveolar space. It may take up to 48 hours after initial

trauma to determine extent of injury. Most often diagnosed based on history and suspicion.
- **Diagnosis:** Physical exam may show evidence of hypoxia or inspiratory crackles in severe cases. CXR often lags behind clinical findings and therefore CT is the imaging modality of choice when clinical suspicion warrants.
- **Treatment:** Following diagnosis, treatment is generally supportive in nature with supplemental O_2 in more severe cases.

■ **Vocal Cord Dysfunction**
- **Definition:** Paradoxical adduction of the vocal folds during inhalation with resulting airflow obstruction.
- **Diagnosis:** Mimics EIB. High incidence of coexisting GERD (and EIB in 50% of cases). Rule out environmental allergens (laryngeal irritants); psychogenic and neurogenic causes.
- **Treatment:** Managed according to cause, i.e., behavioral (speech-language pathologist).

■ **Other**
Gastroesophageal reflux disease (GERD) and anxiety/panic attacks should also be considered among the differential for dyspnea in the athlete.

GASTROINTESTINAL

■ **Gastroesophageal Reflux Disease (GERD)**
- **Definition:** Multifactorial causes. Increased acid production, lower esophageal sphincter relaxation, increased age, BMI all are considered possible contributions. Athletes have increase in abdominal pressure and decrease in GI blood flow that may predispose to reflux.
- **Diagnosis:** Retrosternal pain that is associated within 1 to 2 hours of eating. GERD can be worse with lying on right side, leaning forward, spicy and fatty foods. Intensity varies but is a significant cause of chest pain. Resolution of pain with antacid or proton pump inhibitor (PPI) is a valid diagnostic option that can save money and time. However, ambulatory pH testing or upper GI endoscopy are also valid options and necessary if blood or swallowing difficulties.
- **Treatment:** Lifestyle modifications for the athlete such as no vigorous exercise within 3 hours of eating and weight loss can be beneficial. Also, dietary medications such as decreased spicy and fatty foods, less caffeine, and mint can be helpful. Otherwise, PPI, H2 antagonists, and promotility agents are utilized.

■ **Hepatic Rupture**
- **Definition:** Due to blunt abdominal trauma. Hepatic injuries are less likely to result in significant bleeds. Hepatomegaly might or might not increase risk for rupture.

- **Diagnosis:** Symptoms include RUQ pain along with radiation to right shoulder. Tenderness to palpation will be present in RUQ. Always check for rebound, guarding, or other peritoneal signs. Hypotension and tachycardia may be present. CT is the gold standard for diagnosis.
- **Treatment:** Hepatic injuries are usually managed conservatively because most are hemodynamically stable. Penetrating liver injuries usually require surgery. An athlete must be hemodynamically stable and pain free before RTP. A repeat CT should be done to document healing.

■ Peptic Ulcer Disease

- **Definition:** Injury or erosions of the mucosal lining due to acid or lack of protective chemicals. *Helicobacter pylori* causes a weakening of protective mucus layer in GI tract. NSAIDs are a very common cause of peptic ulcer disease as they inhibit prostaglandin production.
- **Diagnosis:** Deep burning epigastric pain chronologically associated with eating. May be associated with nausea, vomiting or bloating sensation. Occasionally, may present with hematemesis. May be seen in fatigued athlete. *H. pylori* can be diagnosed by a simple blood test in clinic. If more testing is needed, breath test or biopsy from upper endoscopy can be done. History of NSAID use can also be helpful. CBC can be ordered if blood loss is an issue.
- **Treatment:** *H. pylori* is treated with multiple antibiotics and a proton pump inhibitor. After a treatment regimen, a stool test for *H. pylori* antigen should be done for resolution. Cessation of NSAIDs or addition of a PPI can usually treat the active athlete.

■ Runner's Diarrhea

- **Definition:** Lower GI symptoms including cramping, fecal urgency, frequent loose bowel movements, and incontinence during or after a run.
- **Diagnosis:** Unclear but may be related to autonomic nervous system: increased parasympathetic output or increased sympathetic tone or colonic irritability; ischemic enteropathy from decreased splanchnic blood flow. This occurs with increases in training mileage or intensity or in competition.
- **Treatment:** Reduction in training intensity and duration for 1 to 2 weeks and gradual return to training. May cross-train to maintain aerobic capacity
  - Avoid eating at least 2 hours prior to running.
  - Dietary or fluid triggers should be eliminated: avoid high-fat foods before running; limit caffeine 3 to 6 hours before running (stimulates bowel); low fiber diet may be helpful
  - Anti-diarrhea medications should be used cautiously: Loperamide generally safe. Diphenoxylate hydrochloride and atropine sulfate may have secondary effect on sweating and increase risk of heat injury.
  - May require additional workup with GI consult for unresolving symptoms or "red flag" symptoms.

■ **Side Stitch**
- **Definition:** Intense stabbing or aching pain usually in the RUQ. Typically seen in runners; often seen in deconditioned individuals or in athletes intensifying training, or postprandial exercise. Etiology is unclear. May be related to hypoxia-induced diaphragm muscle spasm, hepatic irritation, adhesions, gas pain or ligamentous stretch.
- **Treatment:** Usually improves with improved conditioning. Avoiding exercise after eating, temporarily ceasing exercise, pacing — start with slow warm up, stretching the right arm over the head and forcefully exhaling through pursed lips can often improve symptoms. Ensure adequate hydration

■ **Splenic Rupture**
- **Definition:** Most common solid organ injury in sport from any form of blunt, high-velocity trauma. Associated with infectious mononucleosis (IM). Will see splenic enlargement in 50% of all cases of IM.
- **Diagnosis:** LUQ pain. Patient may also notice pain in right shoulder (Kehr sign). Tenderness to palpation will be present in LUQ. Always check for rebound, guarding, or other peritoneal signs. Hypotension and tachycardia may be present. CT is the gold standard for diagnosis.
- **Treatment:** Splenic injuries graded from I to V with findings ranging from capsular tears of <1 cm to shattered spleens. Hemodynamic stability and monitoring is the key to on-field management and referral decisions. Also, peritoneal signs require surgery. Serial CT scans are required to document healing and to determine RTP.

GENITOURINARY

■ **Acute Renal Failure**
- **Definition:** Renal failure in athletes is not uncommon and can present with non-specific symptoms. The athletic population is at increased risk due to possible dehydration along with consistent or abused NSAID use. Renal blood flow also decreases with prolonged exercise. Myoglobinuria can also cause renal failure. No symptoms are specific to acute renal failure. Malaise, fatigue, decreased exercise performance, nausea may all be possible. Clinician must have a high index of suspicion.
- **Diagnosis:** Confirmed by basic metabolic profile (BMP). UA may be helpful to check for other possible etiologies. A full history of fluid intake, medication use including herbals, and pattern of urination is required.
- **Treatment:** Cessation of any offending agents is required along with vigorous hydration. Repeat BMP is required. Hospitalization necessary only if patient is ill and unable to properly hydrate.

■ **Exercise-Induced Hematuria**
- **Definition:** Micro- or macroscopic in nature. Hematuria has a long differential diagnosis. Seen more in distance events including swimmers. Symptoms typically not associated with pain. Athlete will notice

hematuria that begins with strenuous activity and resolves with rest. A patient who develops hematuria after trauma should receive more workup. Any signs associated with fever, discharge, pain with urination, weight loss or gain, or pain should also receive a full workup.

- **Diagnosis:** Confirmed by unremarkable history and a normal physical examination along with UA with only blood noted. May be confirmed by urine microscopy.
- **Treatment:** Stop activity for 48 to 72 hours and repeat UA. Some hypothesize that hematuria is a consequence of rapid increase in exercise. A slower increase in training might prevent this problem. If the UA is abnormal after rest, then a full workup is warranted.

Kidney Injuries

- **Definition:** Kidney injury in sport is the most common GU issue, but much less common than splenic injury. A kidney injury results from direct blow to abdomen or flank. Patient will report flank pain and hematuria. May also report bruising, nausea.
- **Diagnosis:** Flank ecchymosis can be seen, such as Grey-Turner sign, which indicates retro-peritoneal bleed. Blood in urine can also be helpful, but should always be confirmed by microscopy. CT is the gold standard for diagnosis.
- **Treatment:** Dictated by a grading scale from 0 to 5 with 5 being the worst and indicating a vascular pedicle injury and hypovolemic shock. Initial therapy is dictated by hemodynamic stability. Grades 1 to 3 can be treated with observation. RTP decision is based on no hematuria and possibly following CT for signs of improvement.

Scrotal Masses

- **Definition:** Wide differential diagnosis, including varicocele, spermatocele, hydrocele, and hematocele. Varicocele exam reveals a "bag of worms" and is left sided 80% to 90% of the time. Testicular cancer is the most common malignancy of teens and males in their twenties. Symptoms vary with the possible diagnosis. Most report insidious onset with little pain. Varicoceles, spermatoceles, and hydroceles can be painful.
- **Diagnosis:** Exam will reveal a "bag of worms" for a varicocele. A hydrocele will trans-illuminate, while a hematocele will not. A solid mass that is separate from the cord and epididymis requires ultrasound or possible surgical exploration.
- **Treatment:** Treatment depends upon diagnosis. Most that are painful are treated with pain control and increased support. A varicocele may be associated with infertility and may require surgical intervention. Cancer requires immediate urologic referral.

Testicular Torsion

- **Definition:** Injury to the blood supply and spermatic cord is most common in the adolescent age group. This is considered a urologic emergency as irreversible damage can take place in a short time. An adolescent male with unilateral testicular pain has testicular torsion until proven

otherwise. Patient may or may not report a history of trauma along with unilateral swelling and significant pain. May be associated with nausea, vomiting.
- **Diagnosis:** Unilateral scrotal edema noted along with induration of the scrotal skin. May have a high riding testicle along with absence of the cremasteric reflex. This reflex is tested by rubbing the inner ipsilateral thigh and is considered absent when the hemiscrotum will not rise. Elevation of the scrotum may relieve the pain with epididymitis but worsen the pain with testicular torsion. A Doppler ultrasound should be done but should not delay surgical intervention.
- **Treatment:** Manual reduction of the torsion may be attempted after a cord block but should not delay surgical treatment. The optimum treatment time is within 6 hours.

■ **Torsion of the Appendix Testes**
- **Definition:** Has same risk factors as testicular torsion injury but affects only the appendix of the testicle. The symptoms of torsion of the appendix testes are similar to the symptoms associated with testicular torsion.
- **Diagnosis:** Exam will reveal a possible "blue dot" sign, which is a small lump that appears over the superior pole of the testicle when the skin is pulled tight over it. US can confirm the diagnosis.
- **Treatment:** Treatment is conservative with pain coverage and follow up as needed. The necrosis associated with the torsion is not damaging to surrounding tissue. May reduce activity and increase scrotal support.

■ **Urethral and Bladder Injury**
- **Definition:** Both injuries are related to significant trauma. Typically bladder injury is related with a full or distended bladder. Each injury is associated with hematuria and blood from the urethral meatus. For a urethral tear, a high-riding or absent prostate.
- **Diagnosis:** Typically made by history and physical examination findings. A retrograde urethrogram or cystoscopy will confirm the diagnosis. Always include possible fractures in the pelvis and lumbar spine as urethral and bladder injuries are associated with fractures.
- **Treatment:** Obvious peritoneal signs are a surgical emergency; transport to appropriate facility. In all cases, urologic consult is required as urethral and bladder injuries require frequent urinalysis and possible stent or catheter placement to allow healing.

DERMATOLOGIC

■ **Dermatophytes (General)**
- **Definition:** Fungi that require keratin for growth and therefore cause superficial infections of the skin, hair, and nails. Transmission is via direct contact with infected individuals, animals, and soil or indirectly

through items contaminated with fomites. *Microsporum, Trichophyton,* and *Epidermophyton* species.

- **Diagnosis:** Distinct erythematous, scaly, and often raised border due to an inflammatory response with central clearing. Clinical appearance and hyphae on KOH microscopy. Occasionally Wood lamp or culture is needed.
- **Treatment:** Topical antifungal. Fungicidal allylamines are faster with higher cure rate (e.g., naftifine, terbinafine). Fungistatic azoles (e.g., clotrimazole, econazole, ketoconazole, miconazole). Oral antifungal for tinea capitis (griseofulvin) and barbae and onychomycosis (itraconazole, fluconazole, terbinafine).

■ **Folliculitis**
- **Definition:** Inflammation of hair follicle(s). Follicles are damaged by friction from clothing, blockage of the follicle, or shaving, which leads to infection with *Staphylococcus aureus* (common) or pseudomonas (hot tub).
- **Diagnosis:** Erythematous rash with/without central pustule at hair follicle. Lesions usually cluster in groups. Often pruritic. Lesions may crust over.
- **Treatment:** Warm saline compresses t.i.d. Topical antibiotics (Bactroban, Bacitracin). Shaving should be avoided in involved areas. Topical antifungal agents should be considered in select patients. Oral antibiotics for persistence or extensive disease. Consider monthly Bactroban to nares bid for 5 days per month to reduce *S. aureus* colonization.
- **RTP:** *NCAA Wrestling Guidelines:* No new skin lesions for 48 hours before meet. Must have completed 72 hours of antibiotic therapy. No moist or draining lesions at meet time. Cannot cover active bacterial lesions to allow participation.

■ **Herpes Simplex Virus**
- **Definition:** Cluster of painful vesicles on an erythematous base. Two types:
  - *Type 1:* Generally oral/skin
    - Herpes gladiatorum
    - Cold sores
  - *Type 2:* Generally genital

  Transmission: Skin to skin. Viral shedding can occur in absence of lesions. Permanent infection remains dormant in dorsal root ganglion and can emerge with stress.
- **Diagnosis:** Clinical based on vesicular rash appearance. Can confirm with viral culture or PCR.
- **Treatment:** Antiviral (acyclovir, famciclovir, valacyclovir) to reduce shedding. Acyclovir: 400 mg 3 to 5 times/day for 5 to 7 days at onset of prodrome. May use topical anesthetic for oral lesions. Oral opiates reserved for severe cases.

- **RTP:** *NCAA Wrestling Guidelines*: No systemic symptoms. No new lesions for 72 hours. Existing lesions must have firm adherent crust. Prescription therapy for 120 hours.

■ Impetigo
- **Definition:** Highly contagious bacterial infection caused by beta-hemolytic *Streptococcus* more than *Staphylococcus*.
- **Diagnosis:** Serosanguinous, honey-crusted pustules on erythematous base. May be painful.
- **Treatment:** Mupirocin ointment t.i.d. with/without oral antibiotics (Erythro/Azithro-mycin, Dicloxacillin, Keflex) for 10 days.
- **RTP:** *NCAA Wrestling Guidelines*: See Folliculitis guidelines.

■ Molluscum Contagiosum
- **Definition:.** Caused by pox virus. Highly contagious; spread via skin contact to others or self, water, equipment, towels. Self-limited, resolving over weeks and up to months without treatment.
- **Diagnosis:** Small, umbilicated flesh-colored, dome-shaped papules
- **Treatment:** Liquid N2, cantharidin, electrocautery, imiquimod 5% (Aldara), tretinoin (Retin-A).
- **RTP:** *NCAA Wrestling Guidelines*: Curette or remove lesions prior to meet, then cover with gas-permeable membrane followed by stretch tape.

■ Pitted Keratolysis
- **Definition:** Plaque with pits of variable depth on weight-bearing plantar surfaces. Caused by hyperhidrosis (sweat) and bacteria.
- **Diagnosis:** Pungent foot odor. Generally non-tender.
- **Treatment:** Topical antibiotic bid for 2 to 4 weeks. Proper footwear (fitting and non-occlusive) including absorbent cotton socks changed frequently and wicking socks. Roll-on antiperspirant (↓hyperhidrosis).
- **Prevention:** Topical foot powder (Drysol). Good foot hygiene.

■ Tinea Corporis
- **Definition:** Fungal infection of the body (caused by *Trichophyton* species).
- **Diagnosis:** Papulosquamous lesions with sharply demarcated red borders and central clearing. Itching and pain.
- **Treatment:** Topical antifungal bid until resolved. Oral antifungal: ketaconazole 200 mg for 1 to 2 weeks, terbinafine 250 mg for 1 to 2 weeks.
- **RTP:** *NCAA Wrestling Guidelines*: Topical antifungal for 72 hours. Coverage of lesions with gas-permeable dressing and stretch tape. Minimum of 2 weeks of systemic antifungal therapy for scalp lesions. Wrestlers with extensive lesions are disqualified.

■ Tinea Pedis
- **Definition:** Fungal infection of the sole of the foot and web spaces caused by *Trichophyton* or *Epidermophyton* species.
- **Diagnosis:** Itchy, burning, red, scaly or flaky rash. Cracking of skin between the toes.

- **Treatment:** Topical antifungal creams or sprays. Foot powder. Clears in about 2 to 4 weeks. Use antibacterial soap to wash feet. Dry feet thoroughly after showering and swimming. Disinfect showers and bathtubs with bleach every week. Do not wear wet socks. Avoid sharing towels, shoes, or sandals.

■ **Tinea Versicolor**
- **Definition:** Fungal infection of skin caused by *Malassezia furfur.*
- **Diagnosis:** Chronic, asymptomatic pigmented and scaly patch or macules. Darker on light skin and lighter on dark skin. Rash can be more apparent with exercise or sun tanning. Can be pruritic with sweating during exercise. Wood lamp (black light): yellow-green fluorescence.
- **Symptoms:** Spaghetti and meatballs appearance on KOH scraping.
- **Treatment:**
  - Topical antifungal for 30 minutes for 5 to 10 days or overnight (rinse next day).
    - 2.5% Selenium sulfide (Selsun shampoo).
    - Ketoconazole shampoo to skin.
  - Oral antifungal:
    - Ketoconazole
    - Exercise with sweating for 1 hour after dose to get medicine to hair root.

■ **Veruca Vulgaris (Common Wart)**
- **Definition:** Small non-tender wart caused by HPV infecting the epidermis. Transmitted through direct contact and through shared clothing, especially through open cuts in the skin. Existing warts can shed HPV, which can lead to new warts. Small black dots are thrombosed capillaries in hyperkeratotic skin. Self-limited, but may take years.
- **Diagnosis:** Flesh-colored, soft or scaling papule or nodule
- **Treatment:** Create inflammation
  - Salicylic acid with/without 40% plaster compound (Mediplast) with occlusion
  - Liquid N 2
  - Electrocautery
  - Duct tape
  - Dinitrochlorobenzene (DNCB)
- **RTP:** *NCAA Wrestling Guidelines:* Multiple digitate verrucae on face must be covered by mask or disqualification. Solitary lesions can be curetted and covered.

FEMALE ATHLETE

■ **Exercise and Pregnancy**
- There is no evidence that non-contact exercise has a detrimental effect on pregnancy or labor or fetal well being.
- In the absence of contraindications, pregnant women should be encouraged to engage in regular, moderate-intensity physical activity.

- Exercise during pregnancy may make pregnancy more comfortable, shorten labor, and require less need for intervention during delivery.
- Avoid supine position as much as possible and very hot or humid weather.
- Specific recommendations against scuba diving and sports at risk for abdominal trauma.
- There are no definitive guidelines for elite or endurance athletes during pregnancy.
- Target HR concept abandoned by ACOG.

ACOG CONTRAINDICATIONS TO EXERCISE DURING PREGNANCY (1994)*

◼ Absolute Contraindications to Aerobic Exercise during Pregnancy
- Hemodynamically significant heart disease
- Restrictive lung disease
- Incompetent cervix/cerclage
- Multiple gestation at risk for premature labor
- Persistent 2nd or 3rd trimester bleeding
- Placenta previa after 26 weeks
- Premature labor during the current pregnancy
- Ruptured membranes
- Preeclampsia/pregnancy-induced HTN

◼ Relative Contraindications to Aerobic Exercise during Pregnancy
- Severe anemia
- Unevaluated maternal cardiac arrhythmia
- Chronic bronchitis
- Poorly controlled type 1 DM
- Extreme morbid obesity
- Extreme underweight (BMI <12)
- History of extremely sedentary lifestyle
- IUGR in current pregnancy
- Poorly controlled HTN
- Orthopedic limitations
- Poorly controlled seizure disorder
- Heavy smoker

◼ Warning Signs to Terminate Exercise while Pregnant
- Vaginal bleeding
- Dyspnea prior to exertion
- Dizziness
- Headache
- Chest pain
- Muscle weakness
- Calf pain or swelling (need to rule out thrombophelbitis)

*American College of Obstetricians and Gynecologist Exercise during pregnancy and the postpartum period: ACOG Committee Opinion No. 267. Obstet Gynecol 99(1):171-73, 2002; O'Conner, Sports Medicine, Just the Facts: 2005.

- Preterm labor
- Decreased fetal movement
- Amniotic fluid leakage

■ Female Athlete Triad (FAT)

Most common in sports that focus on weight (gymnastics, dance, distance running). Associated with declining performance and increased injury. Weight <85% of expected for height and age. Evaluate and screen for at risk athletes.

- **Three Components**: Disordered eating, amenorrhea, and osteoporosis.

  Disordered Eating:
  - Spectrum from calorie restriction to classic eating disorders (anorexia nervosa and bulimia).
  - Female athletes at higher risk than general population (15% to 62% of college athletes report history of eating disorder).

  Amenorrhea:
  - Menstrual dysfunction 2 to 3 times more common in athlete vs. non-athlete.
  - Etiology: multi-factorial, including body weight and composition, training, nutrition, psychosocial factors.
  - "Energy drain hypothesis": Inadequate stored energy and inadequate intake relative to energy expenditure. Brain perceives menstrual blood loss as further energy loss and disrupts HPO axis.

  Osteopenia:
  - *Osteopenia*: 1 to 2.5 SD below young adult mean BMD.
  - *Osteoporosis*: Greater than 2.5 SD below young adult BMD.
  - Amenorrheic hypoestrogenic athlete at risk for osteoporosis and stress fractures
  - Consider DEXA if amenorrhea for more than 6 months or if there is prolonged oligomenorrhea.

- **Treatment:** Coordinated team approach with coach, parent, ATC, nutritionist, psychiatrist, and physician. Restore normal menstrual cycle, HRT, optimize nutrition and prescribe antidepressants. Vitamin supplements of iron and calcium (1,500 mg q.d.) and vitamin D (400 to 800 IU q.d.). Menses will resume at approximately 90% of ideal body weight.

HEMATOLOGY

■ Athletic Pseudoanemia

- **Definition:** Endurance training increased both the plasma volume and RBC production. Plasma expansion exceeds the increase in RBC production causing a dilutional reduction in Hgb/Hct. Not a true anemia but a physiologic adaptation that promotes increased CO and O_2 delivery; protects against hyperviscosity. Hemodilution of conditioning can reverse within days of terminating endurance training.

- **Diagnosis:** should have normal RBC indices, reticulocyte count, and serum ferritin.

Condition reversed when testing after several days of rest.

■ Anemia from Blood Loss

- **Exercise associated GI blood loss:**
  - Typically with endurance events and usually minor.
  - Transient ischemia or mechanical contusion (e.g., cecal slap syndrome).
  - Must rule out more serious pathology if warranted.
- **Menstrual blood loss:**
  - Menstrual flow and iron replacement should be considered when evaluating a female for anemia.
  - Treatment is focused on reducing excessive or prolonged bleeding and compensating for iron losses.
- **Exertional hemolysis:**
  - Intravascular destruction of RBCs with exertional activity.
  - Typically not significant enough to affect RBC parameters.
  - Seen in runners; less so in swimmers and weight lifters.
  - Intravascular turbulence, acidosis, elevated temperature in the muscle tissue may be the cause.
  - Labs: Reticulocyte count, RDW, and MCV may be elevated

■ Iron Deficiency Anemia

- **Definition:** Most common nutritional deficit in the United States and most common cause of true anemia in the athlete and non-athlete. Incidence greater in females from menstrual losses (or from decreased or inadequate PO intake).
- **Diagnosis:** Low Hgb and Hct with low MCV and MCH with/without RDW. Low serum ferritin levels, TIBC elevated.
- **Treatment:** Iron replacement 325 mg up to TID with vitamin C to improve absorption; dietician consult. Endurance improves with elevated ferritin levels.

■ Sickle Cell Trait (SCT)

- **Definition:** Genetic abnormality of RBCs causing an irregular shape and sickling of all RBCs; Hgb S is present with Hgb A in RBCs. Present in 8% of blacks in the United States.
  - Typically has little impairment on athletic performance although there may be higher risk of complications with exercise at altitude or dehydration.
  - Sequelae include rhabdomyolysis, splenic syndrome, tissue necrosis, renal deficiency and sudden death.
- **Clinical symptoms**: Muscle cramping, fatigue (greater risk in heat stress environments).
- **Tests:** Blood test for heterozygous presence of HbA and S in SST; microscopic hematuria.
- **Treatment:** Hydration, acclimatization, modifying and monitoring activities.

NEUROLOGIC

■ Axillary Nerve Injury

- **Anatomy:** C5-C6 nerve roots from posterior cord. Passes through quadrilateral space and divides into anterior and posterior trunks. Anterior trunk innervates anterior and medial deltoid. Posterior trunk innervates posterior deltoid, teres minor, and ends as arm lateral cutaneous nerve.
- **Definition:** Blunt shoulder injury/shoulder dislocations, humeral fractures, quadrilateral space syndrome.
- **Diagnosis:** May have posterior shoulder pain and parasthesias. Deltoid weakness in one or all regions. Sensory loss circumferentially at upper lateral arm. Pain exacerbated with shoulder abduction and/or external rotation. May need EMG studies.
- **Treatment:** Rest acutely. Physical therapy with ROM and passive shoulder exercises progressing to resistive motion/strengthening. Consider surgical exploration if no improvement in 3 to 6 months.

■ Burners/Stingers

- **Anatomy:** No single specific nerve injury, however, typically upper/medial trunk of brachial plexus and associated peripheral nerves.
- **Definition:** Typically secondary to traction injuries of the neck or shoulder abduction/extension injuries. At risk are participants in collision sports (football) and wrestlers.
- **Diagnosis:** Sharp, burning pain and dysthesias radiating from the supraclavicular region extending distally down the arm. Symptoms typically last seconds to minutes and may be followed with transient motor weakness of shoulder external rotators or bicep curl. Complete neuromuscular exam to rule out serious injury. Results of exam may vary from normal exam to numbness/weakness in specific nerve(s) injured. Common are suprascapular and musculocutaneous nerves.
- **Treatment:** No direct treatment. Symptoms typically resolve spontaneously. Treatment should focus on recurrence prevention. This can be done with padding, improved technique (tackling), and proper conditioning program. If weakness last >3 weeks, consider EMG/NCV. RTP should be based upon normal strength and ROM. EMG may be abnormal for >1 year in spite of no symptoms.

■ Long Thoracic Nerve Injury

- **Anatomy:** C5-C7 nerve roots. Purely motor nerve which lies deep to clavicle and brachial plexus and innervates serratus anterior along anterolateral chest wall.
- **Definition:** Blunt or recurrent trauma, surgical positioning. Less commonly can occur with compression/entrapment injuries. May also be caused by a viral upper respiratory illness (Parsonage-Turner syndrome).
- **Diagnosis:** Scapular winging while standing with arms at side (inferior scapular angle translocated medially) or with shoulder protraction. May have a dull ache about shoulder. Winging exacerbated with push up

against wall. Be sure to differentiate winging from dorsal scapular nerve injury (rhomboids) or spinal accessory nerve injury (trapezius).
- **Treatment:** Limit further injury by limiting overhead activities. Shoulder physical therapy focusing on rhomboids, trapezius, pectoralis muscles. Nerve function usually recovers completely and normal function may take as long as 18 months. RTP as pain permits.

Median Nerve Injury
- **Anatomy:** C6-T1 nerve roots. Innervates the pronator teres/quadrates. Palmaris longus, forearm flexors, thenar muscles and lumbricals. Provides sensation to lateral palmar surface and digits 1 to 3 and ½ of digit 4.
- **Definition:** Repetitive activities, space occupying lesions. Multiple entrapment sites along the course of the nerve at the elbow and forearm with the most common being the carpal tunnel. Possible entrapment sites: ligament of Struthers, pronator syndrome, anterior interosseous nerve syndrome, carpal tunnel syndrome, digital nerve entrapment.
- **Diagnosis:** Tingling, numbness, weakness in median nerve distribution. Severity and distribution of neurological symptoms vary depending on proximity of lesion/compression. Numbness and weakness depending on proximity of injury. Special considerations include:
  - *Pronator syndrome*: Pain on active resistive forearm pronation, positive Tinel sign, negative Phalen maneuver.
  - *Anterior interosseous nerve syndrome*: Purely motor, positive "O" sign (inability to hold an ok sign).
  - *Carpal tunnel*: Nocturnal numbness, positive Phalen maneuver, positive Tinel sign, sensory deficit in nerve distribution.
- **Treatment:** Conservative treatment including rest, splinting, NSAIDs, avoidance of repetitive/aggravating activity, and possible steroid injection. Surgical release reserved for non-improving cases.

Musculocutaneous Nerve Injury
- **Anatomy:** C5-C7 nerve roots from lateral cord. Innervates coracobrachialis, brachialis, and biceps brachii muscles then ends as forearm lateral cutaneous nerve.
- **Definition:** Uncommon. Possible injury with shoulder dislocation. May have sensory entrapment at elbow with strongly resisted extension and pronation of elbow.
- **Diagnosis:** Biceps, brachialis weakness. Lateral forearm numbness or pain. Weakness with elbow flexion (active/passive), positive Tinel sign at elbow, possible decreased biceps reflex.
- **Treatment:** Rest, avoid high resistance exercises or excessive traction on muscles. PT focusing on gentle stretching and ROM initially and progressing to strengthening. NSAIDs. Sensory entrapment at elbow may require surgical decompression.

Radial Nerve Injury
- **Anatomy:** C5-C8 nerve roots. Innervates triceps in arm and anconeus, brachioradialis, supinator, abductor pollicis longus and extensors in

forearm. Provides sensation to dorsal arm/forearm, dorsum of lateral hand, first web space and digits 1 to 3 proximal phalanges.

- **Definition:** May suffer from proximal entrapment; humerus fracture, improper use of crutches, Saturday night compression/palsy or distal entrapment at elbow; repetitive motion or space occupying lesions.
- **Diagnosis:** Wrist drop, elbow flexion weakness. May have pain/numbness in sensory distribution. Proximal entrapment: slight weakness in elbow flexion (brachioradialis) possible. Decreased triceps weakness and loss of reflex. May also include distal entrapment signs/symptoms. Distal entrapment: No sensory deficits. Partial wrist drop with radially deviated wrist extension. May need EMG.
- **Treatment:** Most injuries neuropraxic and recover spontaneously in 4 to 5 months with conservative management.

■ Spinal Accessory Nerve Palsy

- **Anatomy:** CN XI (C1-C5) innervates sternocleidomastoid, passes through posterior triangle then innervates trapezius. Purely motor.
- **Definition:** Injuries involving percussion/compression of the posterior triangle. Direct blow to shoulder. Shoulder dislocation. Compression from backpack straps. Pain over trapezius exacerbated with movement. Feelings of heaviness in affected arm. Difficulty with overhead activities, heavy lifting, prolonged driving/writing.
- **Diagnosis:** Drooping of affected shoulder, acromion prominence, limited motion in lateral abduction, forward shoulder flexion, and scapular rotation. Test trapezius strength, lateral abduction of arm, 100° to 180° with arm internally rotated and hand pronated. Test SCM by resisted head rotation and head flexion. May need EMG studies. May develop adhesive capsulitis.
- **Treatment:** Most respond to conservative treatment including ROM/strengthening exercises to the shoulder girdle/scapular region. Avoid electrical stimulation initially to prevent overloading regenerating motor units. Surgical treatment with Eden-Lange dynamic muscle transfer.

■ Suprascapular Nerve Injury

- **Anatomy:** C5-C6 nerve roots. Passes through suprascapular notch under transverse scapular ligament and innervates supraspinatus. Continues around scapular spine under spinoglenoid ligament to innervate infraspinatus.
- **Definition:** Two main sites of impingement: at suprascapular notch and at spinoglenoid ligament. Traumatic (scapula fracture)/nontraumatic (overhead loading, backpack straps, cyst) injuries causing compression of nerve at either site of possible entrapment.
- **Diagnosis:** Vague shoulder or AC joint pain. Weakness. May be worse with overhead activities. Weakness and/or atrophy in supra/infraspinatus muscles (abduction/external rotation). May have positive Tinel sign at scapular notch. MRI may diagnosis ganglion or labral cyst at the suprascapular notch and is common in athletes due to underlying shoulder pathology. May need EMG studies.

- **Treatment:** Avoid exacerbating activities. NSAIDs; physical therapy; surgical release may be needed in severe cases.

■ Thoracic Outlet Syndrome
- **Anatomy:** Most commonly secondary to vascular entrapment of subclavian or axillary artery/vein. True neurogenic cause involving the lower trunk of brachial plexus is extremely rare. Postural mechanics is another common cause.
- **Definition:** Presence of a cervical rib or other congenital/structural anomalies. Trauma. Compression/space occupying lesions.
- **Diagnosis:** Palor/cyanosis, vague shoulder/arm pain, muscle fatigue (claudication) common with vascular etiology. Parasthesias in ulnar distribution of hand and forearm common in neurogenic etiology. Symptoms may mimic carpal tunnel. Reproducible symptoms as above. Classic exam tests (Adson test, Wright maneuver) proven to be equivocal with high false positives. X-rays/EMG may aid in diagnosis.
- **Treatment:** Physical therapy emphasizing postural shoulder and scapula biomechanics with stretching of the pec minor and scalenes. Trigger point injections, US, electric stimulation, pain control. Surgical intervention as a last resort.

■ Ulnar Nerve Injury
- **Anatomy:** C8-T1 nerve roots. Innervates flexor digitorum profundus, flexor carpi ulnaris, abductor digiti minimi, intrinsic hand muscles, adductor pollicis and 3rd and 4th lumbricals. It provides sensation to the dorsal, medial surface of the hand.
- **Definition:** Repetitive trauma, overhand/valgus traction injuries, space occupying lesions, trauma/fracture around elbow and tight casts after fracture. Most common site of trauma to nerve is at the elbow or entrapment at Guyon canal at the wrist.
- **Diagnosis:** Severity and distribution of neurologic symptoms vary depending on site of lesion/compression. Common presentation is paresthesias in the 4th and 5th digits. Possible weakness with fine motor activities. Flexion contracture of the PIP (5th digit) or claw hand. Positive elbow flexion test: Exacerbation of symptoms with continuous elbow flexion suggests pathology at elbow. Decreased grip strength. May need EMG to differentiate site of entrapment. Positive Tinel sign at cubital tunnel vs. retrocondylar groove may help differentiate site of elbow entrapment.
- **Treatment:** Conservative management including strengthening or relative rest as indicated initially. If motor weakness is present or symptoms do not improve with time, surgical release may be indicated.

V ■ INFECTIOUS DISEASE

■ **Bronchitis**
- **Definition:** Caused by viral (more common) or bacterial agent.
- **Diagnosis:** Cough for 1 to 2 weeks, increased sputum, fever, nasal congestion, rhinorrhea, pharyngitis, chest congestion, wheezing. Rhonchi often present. Labs are typically non-specific, except leukocytosis with left shift suggests bacterial and marked lymphocytosis suggests pertussis. X-ray is typically negative.
- **Treatment:**
  Viral:
  - Symptomatic and supportive: decongestant, expectorant, cough suppressant, bronchodilator, antipyretics.
  - Influenza treatment if applicable.
  Bacterial:
  - Macrolide or tetracycline for atypicals.
    - First line: Azithromycin 500 mg once and 250 mg for 4 days or erythromycin 500 mg q.d. for 3 days.
    - Second line: Bactrim DS for 14 days.
  - Amoxicillin.

■ **HIV/AIDS**
- **Definition:** A retrovirus that infects helper T cells leading to immunosuppression and AIDS. Adolescents are the fastest growing age group of new infections: unprotected sex, sharing needles. Athletes seen as "high risk" group.
- **Diagnosis:** Symptoms may include acute flu-like illness followed by asymptomatic period during which the virus replicates and antibodies are formed. Can have multiple manifestations with progression to AIDS.
  - **Tests:** HIV: ELISA screening, Western blot confirmation.
- **Treatment:** Pharmacotherapy: Variable combinations of anti-retrovirals.
- **RTP:** No validated reports of transmission in the athletic setting, therefore there is no recommended restriction if an athlete is HIV positive. One court case upheld exclusion of one athlete from contact sport of karate.
- **NCAA Recommendations:** Although sporting transmission is rare (1 per 85 million game contacts in football), remove bloody uniforms and cover open wounds before RTP. Take standard precautions.
- **Exercise:**
  HIV: Full exercise as tolerated:
  - Increases LBM
  - Associated with slower progression to AIDS

AIDS: Limited to moderate exercise as tolerated.
- Participation decisions are made on the basis of the individual's health status.
- No evidence that moderate-intensity activity is harmful; long-term effects of intense training are unknown.

Mononucleosis

- **Definition:** Viral infection caused by the Epstein-Barr virus (majority of cases) from salivary contact; incubation 30 to 50 days; peak incidence 15 to 21 year olds (1% to 3% of college students yearly). There is no evidence that IM is more or less prevalent in student-athlete population
- **Diagnosis:** Fever, fatigue, malaise, anorexia, exudative tonsillopharyngitis, tender posterior lymphandenopathy is often a first clue; splenomegaly.
  - Deterioration of athletic performance may be only presenting symptom
  - *Labs:* Mild LFT elevation, atypical lymphocytosis, heterophile antibodies.
  - Monospot (heterophile antibodies) may be falsely negative in 50% of cases within the first 7 to 10 days. False negative rate as high as 15% even after 3 weeks.
  - *Serologies:*
    - EBV: anti-VCA IgM (acute) and IgG (acute and chronic); anti-EBNA: acute (-), chronic (+).
    - CMV: IgM (acute) and IgG (chronic).
  - Splenomegaly in IM is nearly universal but splenic rupture is rare.
  - Spleen most vulnerable to rupture in the first 3 to 4 weeks of illness; ruptures beyond this timeframe are extremely rare.
  - Physical exam for splenic enlargement not sensitive (found on 17% of exams and 100% on US, which is the preferred modality for imaging spleen).
  - Mononucleosis, because of the risk of splenic rupture, is a contraindication to participation in contact sports or activity in which trauma or increased abdominal pressure/Valsalva could occur for first 3 weeks of illness.
  - One time imaging for assessment of splenomegaly not recommended due to wide variability in "normal" sizes.
- **Treatment:** Supportive to provide relief with attention to potential complications
  Steroids: controversial; not recommended in uncomplicated cases.
- **RTP:** Lack of consensus.
  - Light, non-contact activities may commence 3 weeks from symptom onset. Often difficult for patients to define the onset of symptoms
  - Afebrile, asymptomatic, and have achieved appropriate level of fitness.
  - Light activity assumes activity will avoid any chest and/or abdominal trauma and Valsalva, until asymptomatic. Risk of contact and/or collision and age of the athlete should be considered

- Inform that risk of spleen rupture is never zero with or without IM, although overwhelming majority of splenic ruptures occur in the first 3 weeks; few reports of rupture beyond 28 days after diagnosis. Decisions should be made on a case-by-case basis recognizing all risk factors.
  - Serial studies should be considered.
  - Most experts agree that vigorous sports be restricted until spleen has returned to normal size and position under the rib cage.

■ Methicillin-Resistant Staphylococcus Aureus (MRSA)

- **Definition:** *S. aureus* infections commonly cause soft tissue and systemic infections . Most are mild and easily treated , but if not detected and treated appropriately some can lead to significant morbidity and mortality. MRSA infections have developed resistance to some common antibiotics and have a disproportionate incidence in the athletic community.
- **Diagnosis:** Pain, redness, swelling and possibly drainage from a wound on the skin. There may be a history of an abrasion or other skin compromise.
  - Concurrent skin conditions (eczema, herpes) are risk factors.
  - Athletes often present for evaluation of a "spider bite"; furuncles, carbuncles, abscesses.
  - Risk factors: turf burns or any soft tissue breaks or lesions, athletes who are shaving, skin-to-skin contact; towel or personal item sharing, poor hygiene, equipment contact.
- **Treatment:** Gold standard: I&D; culture lesions; systemic antibiotic therapy.
  - Non-serious: Oral TMP/SMX or doxycycline.
  - Serious outpatient: Oral clindamycin or TMP/SMX + rifampin.
  - Serious in patient: IV clindamycin or vancomycin.
  - Life threatening: Vancomycin with/without nafcillin.
  - Promote good hygiene and clean facilities used by trainers, coaches, parents, and players. Hand hygiene is the single most effective way to reduce MRSA transmission.
- **RTP:** 72 hours in mild-to-moderate skin infections after therapy initiated and no new lesions for 48 hours and clinical improvement is noted. No participation until cleared. Cover lesions with regular wound and dressing checks during competition. Dressing may be removed when lesion has firm adherent crust and all signs of infection have resolved. Athletes should report any suspicious lesions to the ATC or team physician.

■ Pharyngitis

- **Definition:** Sore throat caused by viral (more common) or bacterial agent.
- **Diagnosis:** *Viral:* fever, swollen glands/tonsils, conjunctivitis, cough. *Bacterial:* fever, swollen tender glands, exudative tonsils, no cough. Rapid strep test. Culture as indicated.

- **Treatment:** Warm salt water gargles, humidified air, throat lozenges, analgesics, antipyretics; 10 day course of antibiotics if bacterial source. Penicillin treatment of choice. Alternatives: amoxicillin, cephalosporins, macrolides, clindamycin. Antibiotics render patient non-infectious after 24 hours and protect against rheumatic fever.

Streptococcal Scoring System	
Criteria	**Points**
Temperature >38°C	1
No cough	1
Tender anterior cervical nodes	1
Tonsillar swelling or exudate	1
Age 3 to 14 years	1
Age 15 to 44 years	0
Age >45 years	−1

Total Score	Chance of Infection (%)	Suggested Management	Score	PPV for (+) Throat Culture
0	2 to 3	No culture or antibiotic	1	N/A
1	4 to 6	No culture or antibiotic	2	24%
2	10 to 12	Culture all; treat only if culture (+)	3	22%
3	27 to 28	Culture all; treat only if culture (+)	4	41%
4	38 to 63	Culture all; treat with antibiotics on clinical grounds	5	59%

Upper Respiratory Infection (URI)

- **Definition:** Most common respiratory infection, with rhinovirus the most common agent.
- **Diagnosis:** Malaise, chills, dry scratchy throat, nasal congestion, rhinorrhea hoarseness, headache, cough, sneezing, low-grade fever (except flu with rapidly rising fever). Symptoms can be present for up to 10 to 14 days. No testing indicated except possibly for influenza in winter/spring or during epidemic with rapid enzyme immunoassay (EIA)
- **Treatment:** *Symptomatic and supportive:* Decongestants, NSAIDs/Tylenol, nasal irrigation, cough suppressant, expectorant, MDI. *For influenza:* Oseltamivir, amantadine/rimantadine (influenza B treatment and prevention), zanamivir (influenza A and B treatment)
  - Exercise intensity to be individualized More restriction is appropriate if the temperature is >100.5°F, poor PO intake, myalgias and more severe fatigue and malaise. A general principle:
    - As tolerated, if symptoms above the neck.
    - Rest until symptoms below the neck resolve.

VI ■ OVERTRAINING, UNDER-RECOVERY AND OTHER SYNDROMES

■ **Overtraining**
- **Definition:** A maladaptive response to training from extended overload with inadequate recovery resulting in decrements of performance generally lasting more than 2 weeks.
- **Clinical Symptoms:** Fatigue, sleep disorder, overuse injuries, immune dysfunction.
  - *Sympathetic Overtraining:* Early phase. Manifests with increased resting HR and BP, loss of appetite and LBM, irritability, sleep disturbance and fatigue.
  - *Parasympathetic Overtraining:* More chronic and prolonged overtraining. Manifests with low resting HR and BP, sleep disturbance, depressed mood and fatigue.
- **Physical Exam:** Elevated resting HR taken in morning before getting out of bed (usually >10 BPM over baseline), decreased LBM and depressed mood. Otherwise, exam is normal.
- **Etiology:** Effects 5% to 15% of elite athletes at any one time and as much as 2/3 of runners during athletic career. May be more common in amateur athletes and athletes participating in endurance events, such as swimming, cycling, or running. Susceptible athletes include those who are highly motivated and goal oriented.
- **Hypothesized Causes:**
  - *Chronic glycogen depletion:* Chronic nutritional deficiency leading to chronic glycogen depletion with peripheral muscle fatigue and central fatigue. Related to changes in BCAA.
  - *Autonomic imbalance:* Increase in sympathetic activity from stress and overload. Increased catabolism leading to decreased sympathetic intrinsic activity. Chronically elevated catecholamine levels cause a receptor down regulation and fatigue.
  - *Central fatigue hypothesis:* Peripheral fatigue and nutrient depletion lead to the consumption of BCAA; change in BCAA (to a precursor for serotonin) causes central fatigue.
  - *Glutamine hypothesis (immune dysfunction):* Glutamine deficiency from overload training leads to compromised immune system.
  - *Cytokine hypothesis:* Incomplete recovery of tissue damage with overload creates a systemic increase in pro-inflammatory cytokines, which cause CNS fatigue.
- **Workup:** CBC, ESR, CMP, TSH, ferritin, monospot, B-HCG.
  - Prescribe decrease in intensity or absolute rest for 2 weeks, cross train for enjoyment, decrease possible stressors.

- **Prevention:** Individualize training programs. Coaching and supervised training. Cross training. Reasonable goal setting. Relaxation techniques. Sports psychologist.

▨ Delayed-Onset Muscle Soreness (DOMS)

- **Definition:** Temporary pain and soreness resulting from (eccentric) exercise and training. Onset is usually 12 to 48 hours following exercise and may last 3 to 4 days.
- **Etiology:** Secondary to microtrauma, alterations in calcium metabolism and osmotic changes and is part of an adaptation process. Any unaccustomed movement can lead to DOMS.
- **Physical Exam:** Involved muscles are stiff or tender to palpation. Weakness or fatigue of muscles.
- **Treatment:** Condition improves with time. Avoid vigorous activity. RICE. Stretching debated but may feel good. Gentle massage. Acetaminophen or NSAIDs. Low impact exercise to increase blood flow.
  - Becomes less severe or resolves with increases in fitness.
  - Prevention: warm up before next exercise session; easing into the exercise program with slow gradual changes.

▨ Exercise-Associated Hyponatremia (EAH)

- **Definition:** Low serum sodium levels in individuals during or up to 24 hours after prolonged physical activity (usually Na+ <135 mmol/L).
  - In general, the lower the Na+, the more severe the neurologic symptoms; however, numerical value is not a reliable index of clinical severity.
  - Etiology: Predominantly dilutional. Increase in total body water relative to amount of total body exchangeable Na+ caused by overconsumption of fluids in excess of total body fluid losses; AVP secretion is an exacerbating factor in most cases. Excessive Na+ loss has *not* been demonstrated as a primary causative factor.
- **Diagnosis:** *Early:* Bloating, "puffiness," nausea, vomiting, headache, weight gain. *As severity progresses:* Confusion, disorientation, agitation (cerebral edema), seizures, respiratory distress (pulmonary edema), obtundation, coma, death.
- **Treatment:**
  - *Asymptomatic:* Restrict PO fluid intake until onset of urination. IV NS can worsen the degree of hyponatremia.

Risk Factors for EAH	
Athlete Related:	**Event-Related:**
Low body weight	High availability of drinking fluids
Weight gain during exercise	>4 h exercise duration
Slow running or performance pace	Unusually hot environmental conditions
Female sex	Extremely cold temperature
Race inexperience	
Excessive drinking behavior	
Event inexperience	
NSAIDs	

- *Symptomatic*: Onsite IV access. Avoid isotonic or hypotonic fluids; EAH with signs of respiratory insufficiency, confusion, obtundation, nausea and vomiting can be treated with bolus of hypertonic saline (100 mL of 3% NaCl over 10 minutes) to acutely raise the Na+ and decrease brain edema. Has been used to stabilize athlete prior to hospital transfer.
- **Prevention:**
  - Avoid overconsumption of fluids in excess of fluid losses.
  - Aid stations placed at appropriate intervals (stations placed every 5 km associated with absence of EAH in some studies). Race directors may consider pre-race weights as part of race registration to compare as needed.
  - Ensure availability of Na+ analysis to screen for EAH.
  - Use USATF guidelines to estimate sweat losses and fluid replacement.
  - Some studies report less severe EAH with electrolyte-containing drinks.

■ Stress Fractures

- **Definition:** Accelerated bone remodeling in response to repetitive stresses. Can account for 1% to 20% of all injuries seen in sports medicine clinics. Microfractures from repetitive loading forces, increased load vs. muscular forces, or both.
- **Diagnosis:** Local or point tenderness, swelling, pain with ballistic testing or fulcrum testing. May start with pain with weight-bearing activity only, then progress to pain at rest.
- **Risk Factors:** Changes in playing surface, footwear, intensity or duration of training program in prior 2 to 6 weeks. Women are at 1.5 to 3.5 times greater risk. Women with eating disorders, oligomenorrheic and amenorrheic female athletes, smokers, and those with nutritional irregularities are at higher risk. Site of fracture varies from sport to sport.
- **Radiology:** X-rays specific but not sensitive; 2/3 are initially negative and ½ never develop radiographic evidence. Onset of pain precedes positive radiographic findings by up to 2- to 3 months (periosteal thickening; radiolucent "dreaded black lines"). Bone scan is positive 2 to 8 days after symptoms begin and is sensitive, but not very specific. MRI is also very sensitive and more specific than bone scan. In stress fractures, all 3 phases of triple-phase bone scan will be positive.
- **Treatment:** Protect from further damage. Pain control. Reduce activity below threshold for symptoms. Cross training. No weight bearing, immobilization, orthotics, ice, NSAIDs. Gradual return to activity when pain free. Oral contraceptive pills (females). Correction of biomechanical errors.
- **Prevention:** Gradual increase in training load, calcium supplement.

VII ■ ENVIRONMENTAL MEDICINE

■ **Chilblains/Pernio**
- **Definition:** Mild, inflammatory reaction of skin caused by chronic inter-mittent exposure to damp, non-freezing ambient temperatures. The ears, hands, lower legs, and feet are most commonly involved.
- **Diagnosis:** Cutaneous manifestations of localized edema, erythema, and cyanosis appear within 12 hours of acute exposure. Patients complain of pruritis and burning paresthesias. Primarily a disease of women and children. Women with Raynaud phenomenon are at greater risk. Rewarming may produce tender blue nodules that can persist for several days.
- **Treatment:** Treatment is supportive. Affected skin should be rewarmed, gently bandaged, and elevated. Affected areas are more prone to reinjury in future

■ **Frostbite**
- **Definition:** Can occur on any skin surface but usually limited to ears, nose, face, hands, and feet. Also seen in the penis/scrotum of joggers, burn patients after prolonged ice treatments, and skiers/snowmobilers who did not wear protective eyewear and developed a corneal freezing keratitis. *Frostnip* is on a continuum with frostbite but does not result in tissue loss.
- **Diagnosis:** Involved extremity is painful and appears pale from intense vasoconstriction. Symptoms resolve with rewarming. Classified into *superficial* (first and second degree) and *deep injury* (third and fourth degree).
  - *First Degree:* Partial skin freezing, erythema, mild edema, and lack of blisters. Occasional skin desquamation 5 to10 days later. Patient complains of stinging and burning, followed by throbbing. Prognosis is excellent.
  - *Second Degree:* Full-thickness freezing, erythema, moderate edema. Clear fluid blisters filled with thromboxane and prostaglandins form within 6 to 12 hours. Desquamation occurs over days and black eschar forms. Patient complains of numbness, followed by throbbing. Prognosis is good.
  - *Third Degree:* Full-thickness and subcutaneous freezing. Hemorrhagic blisters form and are associated with bluish-gray discoloration of the skin and skin necrosis. Patient initially feels no sensation and states involved extremity feels like "a block of wood." This is followed by burning, shooting pains. Prognosis is poor.
  - *Fourth Degree:* Full-thickness skin, subcutaneous tissue, muscle, tendon, and bone freezing. Very little edema seen. Skin is mottled, nonblanching, and cyanotic. Eventually forms dry, mummified eschar. Patient complains of deep, aching joint pain. Prognosis is very poor.

- **Treatment:** Rapid rewarming is hallmark of therapy. Never rewarm in the field unless definitive care can be established; refreezing can cause further tissue destruction. Avoid further cold injury. Wet constrictive clothing should be removed. Wrap involved extremities in dry gauze and elevate. Separate involved fingers and toes with wrap. Change dressings daily
    - **Thaw:** Use water bath ranging from 40° to 42°C (104° to 107°F) for 10 to 30 minutes with active motion. Parenteral analgesics as needed (Morphine/Demerol). Water that is too hot and dry heat from campfires/heaters can cause further thermal damage to skin.
    - **Post-Thaw:** Clear blisters should be debrided and aspirated; leave hemorrhagic blisters intact. Cover with aloe vera dressings. Tetanus prophylaxis. Regular administration of ibuprofen. Consider penicillin G 500,000 units Q6 hours for 2 to 3 days. Daily hydrotherapy. Hyperbarics if severe and diffuse tissue damage.
- **Prevention:** Adequate clothing that is layered and non-constricting. Proper fitting boots. Cover head and neck because they account for 80% of heat loss. Wear wool and cotton as opposed to synthetic fibers that have poor wicking ability and higher moisture retention. Change out of wet clothes. Avoid smoking, alcohol, and other mental status depressive medications.

■ Trench Foot
- **Definition:** Found in several World War I troops who stood in trenches filled with cold water for prolonged periods of time. Direct soft tissue injury caused by prolonged cooling. Develops slowly over hours to days. Initially reversible but if allowed to progress can become irreversible.
- **Diagnosis:** Initially foot is pale, mottled, anesthetic, pulseless, and immobile. Hyperemic phase begins within hours and is marked with intense burning pain. Reperfusion occurs within 2 to 3 days but anesthesia may persist for weeks or be permanent. In severe cases, tissue sloughing and gangrene may occur.
- **Treatment:** Once early symptoms appear, maximize efforts to rewarm; dry, gently bandage, and elevate feet. Monitor for early signs of infection. Prevention includes staying warm, changing wet socks frequently, proper boot fit, and never sleeping in wet socks or boots.

■ Hypothermia
- **Definition:** Decrease in core body temperature due to heat loss from conduction and convection mechanisms. Body heat loss is greater than in air. Seen in prolonged athletic events where the temperature is below 10°C (50°F) and with increased wind speed and precipitation.
- **Diagnosis:**
    - *Mild:* Core body temperature between 34° and 36°C
    - *Moderate:* Core body temperature between 27° and 34°C
    - *Severe:* Core body temperature below 27°C
  Sign and symptoms include confusion, impaired judgment, shivering, slurred speech, lethargy, disorientation, and paradoxical undressing. May progress to unconsciousness.

- **Treatment:** Prevent further heat loss. Remove wet clothes. Monitor rectal temperature. Active external rewarming with heat packs to groin, axilla, and neck. For severe hypothermia, active internal rewarming with warmed IV fluid, peritoneal lavage, and humidified oxygen. ACLS protocols should be used to follow cardiac monitoring.

HEAT EXPOSURE

■ Heat Cramps
- **Definition:** Occurs in individuals who are sweating and replacing fluid losses with water and other hypotonic solutions. May occur during exercise or after latent period. Nonacclimatized individuals most at risk. Self limited. Believed to be caused by deficiency in sodium, potassium, and fluids.
- **Diagnosis:** Painful, involuntary, spasmodic, contraction of the muscles, most commonly in the calf.
- **Treatment:** Rest in cool place. Fluid and salt replacement either PO or IV.

■ Heat Edema
- **Definition:** Self limited, resolves within days. Caused by cutaneous vasodilation and orthostatic pooling within the extremities. Does not progress to pretibial region. Found most commonly in elderly non-acclimatized individuals who are physically active after prolonged sitting in car, bus, or plane. Also seen in healthy travelers traveling from colder climate.
- **Diagnosis:** Mild swelling of the hands and feet within first few days of exposure to hot environment
- **Treatment:** No specific treatment except elevation and support hose. Diuretics not effective. Predispose to electrolyte abnormalities.

■ Heat Exhaustion
- **Definition:** Heat illness caused by combination of salt and water depletion. No CNS dysfunction. Mental status remains normal.
- **Diagnosis:** Dizziness, light-headedness, nausea, vomiting, headache. Temperature ranges from normal to 40°C (104°F).
- **Treatment:** Rest, volume/electrolyte replacement (PO/IV). Most cases do not require hospitalization.

■ Heat Stroke
- **Definition:** Heat illness cause by salt and water depletion defined by CNS dysfunction and mental status changes. Considered medical emergency; multi-organ system failure.
- **Diagnosis** Temperature >40.5°C (104.9°F). Ataxia may be early sign. Sweating does not exclude diagnosis.
  - *Non-exertional (classic):*
    Occurs during summer heat waves. Common in poor, chronically ill, and extremes of age. Lack of heat dispersion.
  - *Exertional:*
    Consequence of vigorous physical activity. Involves younger population. Increased heat production.

- **Treatment:**
  - ABCs, serial monitoring of core temperature, undress patient.
  - Rapid cooling:
    - Evaporative: spray water on skin blow fans across body
    - Ice packs in groin and axillae
    - Immersion
  - Antipyretics not effective.
  - Stop once core temp reaches 40°C (104°F).

ALTITUDE ILLNESS

▇ Acute Mountain Sickness
- **Diagnosis:** Rapid ascent in unacclimatized person to 2000 meters (6600 feet) or higher. More serious forms of altitude sickness are rarely seen below 2500 meters (8000 feet) and are much more common at very high altitude (3500 meters or 11,500 feet). Symptoms depend on rate of ascent and sleeping altitude.
- **Symptoms:** Initially lightheaded with breathlessness upon exercise. Onset as early as 2 hours, but more typically 8 to 12 hours. Clinical symptoms reported to be similar to "hangover." Bifrontal headache (worse with bending over), fatigue, nausea, vomiting.

▇ High Altitude Cerebral Edema (HACE)
- Most severe form of AMS. Symptoms are ataxia and altered level of consciousness. Coma ensues if no treatment within 12 hours. HA, nausea, and vomiting not always present.
- **Treatment:** Rapid descent. Supplemental O$_2$, steroids, acetazolamide, loop diuretics. Hospital admission for persons remaining ataxic after descent.

▇ High Altitude Pulmonary Edema (HAPE)
- Most lethal of altitude illness. Easily reversible with descent and supplemental O$_2$. Death due to lack of early recognition or inability to descend.
- **Risk Factors:** Exertion, cold, rapid ascent, high salt intake, use of sleeping pills, and prior history.
- **Symptoms:**
  - *Early:* Dry cough, dyspnea with exertion, localized rales, poor exercise performance
  - *Late:* Tachycardia, tachypnea, dyspnea at rest, productive cough, cyanosis, rales. Consciousness worsens as does hypoxia. Worsens at night. More obvious second night at altitude
- **Treatment:** Key is early recognition. Immediate descent, minimize exertion, supplemental O$_2$.

LIGHTNING INJURIES

- **Definition:** Lightning is a direct current that contacts the body and spreads via flashover phenomenon thus usually sparing the deeper organs. Injuries to cardiovascular system and central nervous system are the most devastating. Sports are associated with increased risk. The largest number of injuries and fatalities occur during water sports.

- **Types of Strike**:
  - Direct strike
  - Side flash
  - Contact strike
  - Ground current
  - Stride potential
- **Injuries**:
  - *Cardiovascular Injury*: Current causes direct depolarization of the myocardium with sustained asystole. ECG can show acute injury with ST segment elevations and prolonged QT interval. CK/CK-MB isoenzymes are usually elevated but myocardial infarction is not common.
  - *Neurologic Injury*: Resistance to current is lowest in nervous tissue. Paralysis of medullary respiratory center resulting in respiratory arrest. Heat-induced coagulation of the cortex. Intravascular hemorrhage from head trauma.
  - *Dermatologic Injury*: Ferning burns, flash burns, punctuate burns, contact burns, erythema, blistering and linear streaking.
  - *Otologic Injury*: Ranges from transient hearing loss and vertigo to tympanic rupture.
  - *Ocular Injury*: Cataracts are most common and may occur immediately or 2 years later. Dilated unresponsive pupils may be due to transient autonomic dysfunction and should not be used as sign of brain death. Retinal detachment, retinal hemorrhage, uveitis, hyphema, corneal abrasions also common.
  - *Musculoskeletal Injury*: Extremity fractures, spinal and cervical fractures, compartment syndromes, muscular rupture, and posterior shoulder dislocations.
- **Treatment:** EMS and bystander safety is most important because lightning can strike twice in same place. ABCs (airway, breathing, circulation).
  - *Reverse Triage*: Care for the apparently dead first in multi-casualty lightning strikes. Victims should be transported in full spinal immobilization to tertiary care facility for admission.
- **Prevention:** Remain indoors, seek shelter in a vehicle. If no shelter, head for dense woods or lie in a ditch; avoid open windows and doors; avoid metallic objects; get out of water.
- **NCAA Guidelines:**
  - Designate one individual to monitor weather and to make decision to remove individuals from athletic event/field. Lightning safety plans should be in place ahead of time.
  - Monitor local weather reports daily.
  - Be aware of warning signs of impending storms.
  - Know where the closest safety location is to the field
  - Begin preparation for evacuation if thunderclap heard, suspend activity if lightning seen and head for designated safety locations.

SCUBA/DIVE MEDICINE

■ Arterial Gas Embolism
- **Definition:** Results from gas bubbles entering into the systemic circulation through ruptured pulmonary veins at the terminal bronchiole level. Bubbles pass through the heart and lodge in the small arteries.
- **Diagnosis:** Presents immediately (2 to 10 minutes) after diver surfaces. Sudden LOC within this time period is assumed arterial gas embolism until proven otherwise. Other CNS symptoms include acute stroke symptoms, vertigo, dizziness, or aphasia. Air bubble laden blood returns to the heart causing coronary occlusion and cardiac arrest.
- **Treatment:** Hyperbaric oxygen/recompression therapy effective up to 10 days after event.

■ Barotrauma
Tissue damage from contraction or expansion of gas when pressure in the body is not equal to the ambient pressure.
- **Descent or Squeeze**: Gas is compressed as ambient pressure increases with underwater descent. Ears and sinuses most affected.
- **Ascent or Reverse Squeeze**: Gas is expanded as ambient pressure decreases with ascent. Barodontalgia ("tooth squeeze"), from recent extractions or pulp decay; aerogastralgia ("gas in the gut") from drinking carbonated beverages or eating heavy meals before diving.
- **Pulmonary:** "POPS" (pulmonary over-pressurization syndrome). Diving equipment delivers compressed gas at the same pressure as the environment. Pneumothorax with mediastinal and subcutaneous emphysema occurs if not equilibrated on ascent. Can progress to tension pneumothorax.

■ Decompression Sickness
- **Definition:** Multi-system disorder resulting from gas coming out of solution and forming gas bubbles in blood and body tissues upon ascent. Bubbles form in venous circulation impeding venous return.
- **"The bends":** Refers to the musculoskeletal effects of decompression sickness. Shoulder and elbow joints and spinal cord are most affected. Movement aggravates the pain. Inflation of a BP cuff may relieve the pain over an affected limb.
- **Treatment:** Referred for hyperbaric oxygen/recompression therapy.

■ Nitrogen Narcosis
Nitrogen has an anesthetic effect at elevated partial pressures similar to alcohol. With increasing depth the narcotic effect becomes more apparent.

VIII ■ PAIN MANAGEMENT IN SPORTS MEDICINE

Managing pain is an important aspect of the sports medicine physician's job. The ability to treat acute and chronic pain is a vital skill to possess. The pharmacology of possible drug choices, common side effects, and toxicology will be discussed.

Pharmacologic treatment of pain should begin with identifying the source of pain. Analgesic choice should be directed at the level of pain and titrated to the desired affect while minimizing side effects. Analgesic effect is best treated initially on a scheduled basis. The route of administration should be adjusted as needed to also minimize side effects and maximize analgesia. Depending on the level of pain a non-opioid or opioid should be chosen. Compliance to pharmacotherapy is also important. It is important to note the inverse relationship between frequency of administration and compliance.

Non-opioid analgesics are a first line agent in the treatment of mild to moderate pain. These include topical medications, acetaminophen, NSAIDs, and COX-2 inhibitors. Ultimately, COX-2s are NSAIDs but warrant special mention as each of these medications has its own specific side effects and toxicology. Prescription should take place only after considering the level of pain and the patient's medical history.

Opioid analgesics are often given in combination products. The combination products are excellent treatment for moderate pain associated with acute injuries or post-operatively. Usual combination products have limitations that are associated with the acetaminophen or aspirin in each drug. Short-acting opioids should not be used for chronic pain. Long-acting opioids are excellent for long-term pain management.

NON-OPIOID ANALGESICS

■ Acetaminophen
- May be the first line agent for mild to moderate pain.
- Less effective than full dose NSAIDs but fewer side effects.
- No clinically useful anti-inflammatory, anti-platelet, or adverse GI effects.
- Overdose can cause transient hepatic function test elevations or rarely, fatal hepatic injuries. People who use alcohol or have other hepatic issues can have adverse affects with even minimal doses.
- Normal maximum dose is 4 g per day distributed in 1g q.i.d.

■ NSAIDs
- Most common medication type used in sports medicine. NSAIDs, as a full single dose, have been shown to be as or more effective analgesics than acetaminophen or aspirin.[1]

[1]Abramowicz, M. (ed.). The Medical Letter, Treatment Guidelines from the Medical Letter: Drugs for Pain. Vol. 5 (Issue 56). April 2007.

- Excellent for mild to moderate pain.
- Inhibit cyclooxygenase (COX). Non-selective NSAIDs inhibit COX-1 and COX-2.
  - COX-1 typically aids in the formation of prostaglandins that help protect the gastroduodenal mucosa and support platelet function.
  - COX-2 helps form prostaglandins that mediate inflammation, pain, and fever.

Once again, however:

- NSAIDs should not be used chronically due to the potential for side effects.
- NSAIDs have an analgesic ceiling dose above which there is no more analgesia.
- Aspirin or salicylic acids derivatives have less analgesia than acetaminophen with higher side effects and are therefore not used as much for pain.
- There are 7 families of NSAIDs with traditional thought being that if one medication is not working, switching families might be useful. However, no NSAID has been proven to be more effective with analgesia than another.[2]

  The 7 families:

  1) Salicylates (aspirin, diflunisal)
  2) Acetic acids (indomethacin, etodolac, diclofenac, sulindac, ketorolac)
  3) Propionic acids (ibuprofen, naproxen, ketoprofen)
  4) Pyrazolonic acid (off market)
  5) Fenamic acid (meclofenate)
  6) Naphylalkanones (nabumetone). Has decreased GI symptoms due to preference for COX-2.
  7) Oxicams (meloxicam and piroxicam). Oxicams have a longer half-life.

- **Side Effects:**
  - Anaphylaxis
  - GI bleeding
  - Peptic ulcers and GI perforation
  - Decrease renal blood flow and may lead to fluid retention and possibly hypertension
  - Reversible inhibition of platelet aggregation
  - Aspirin causes irreversible inhibition

▮ COX-2 Inhibitors

- Only celecoxib remains on the market.
- Less GI toxicity than non-selective NSAIDs.
- No advantages regarding kidney functions.
- Does not inhibit platelet function.

---

[2]Davies NM, Skjodt NM. Choosing the right nonsteroidal anti-inflammatory drug for the right patient: a pharmacokinetic approach. Clinical Pharmacokinetics. 2000 May;38(5):377–92.

Pain Management Chart

Medication (Group)	Regular Dose	Maximum Dose	Side Effects	Comments
Acetaminophen	500–1000 mg q4–6 h	4 mg/24 h	Hepatic	Avoid in hepatic failure, alcoholics
Acetylsalicylic acid (ASA)	325–650 mg PO q4 h	5 mg/24 h	Platelet, GI	Irreversible platelet effects
Ibuprofen (Proprionic acid)	600–800 mg q6–8 h	2400 mg /24 h	GI	Usual first line medication
Naprosyn (Proprionic acid)	250–500 mg b.i.d.	1500 mg /24 h	GI	20 times more potent than ASA
Indomethacin (Acetic acid)	IR: 25–75 mg q8–12 h SR: 75 mg b.i.d.	IR: 200 mg/24 h SR: 150 mg/24 h	GI	
Ketorolac (Acetic acid)	30–60 mg IM 10 mg PO t.i.d.	IM: 120 mg IM/24 h PO: 40 mg PO/ 24 h	GI, renal	No more than 5 days of treatment IM or PO
Diclofenac (Acetic acid)	50 mg PO t.i.d.	200 mg/24 h	GI, renal	
Ultram (Tramadol)	50–100 mg PO q4–6	400 mg/24 h	GI, renal	Avoid in opioid dependent, beware with seizure history
Nabumetone (Naphylkanones)	750–1000 mg PO b.i.d.	2000 mg/24 h	GI, renal	Theoretically, less GI side effects
Meloxicam (Oxicam)	7.5 mg PO daily	15 mg/24 h	GI, renal	More potent GI side effects
Piroxicam (Oxicam)	20 mg PO daily	40 mg/24 h	GI, renal	
Celecoxib (COX-2)	200 mg PO daily	400 mg/24 h	Renal	Contraindicated in sulfonamide allergy
Codeine	30–60 mg PO q4 h	600 mg/24 h	Constipation	Use usually limited by acetaminophen
Hydrocodone	5–10 mg PO q4–6 h	1–2 tabs every 4–6 h	Constipation, respiratory	Use usually limited by acetaminophen
Oxycodone	5–10 mg PO q4–6 h	1–2 tabs every 4–6 h	Constipation, respiratory	Use usually limited by acetaminophen

- Rofecoxib (Vioxx) and valdecoxib (Bextra) were voluntarily removed from the market after studies demonstrated a small but statistically significant increase in thrombotic events.

■ **Opioid Analgesics**
- More potent analgesics than most NSAIDs and acetaminophen.
- Effective for moderate to severe pain.
- Have no ceiling for analgesic effect.
- Divided into partial agonists and full agonists.
   * Weak full agonists: Codeine, proproxyphene, hydrocodone, tramadol.
      * Strong full agonists: Morphine, oxycodone, methadone, hydromorphone, fentanyl.
- **Side Effects:** Tolerance and dependence (addictive epotential), constipation, sedation, dizziness, nausea, vomiting, itching, respiratory depression.

IX ■ ATHLETIC DRUG/SUPPLEMENT REFERENCE

- **Definition:** Substances prohibited either in or out of competition.
  - Professional sports, International Olympic Committee (IOC), National Collegiate Athletic Association (NCAA), USA Track and Field (USATF) each have their own testing policies.
  - World Anti-Doping Agency (WADA) prepares and publishes a list used by many groups at the international level.
  - Revised WADA "Prohibited List" International Standard: www.wada-ama.org/en/
  - United States Anti-doping Agency (USADA) is an independent antidoping agency for Olympic sports in the U.S.: www.usantidoping.org
  - NCAA banned list summary: www.ncaa.org/health-safety
  - Examples of PERMITTED Medications: www.usada.org

SUMMARY OF USADA CLASSES AND SUBSTANCES PROHIBITED
In and Out of Competition
- Anabolic agents (e.g., testosterone, DHEA, clenbuterol)
- Hormones and related substances and all releasing factors (e.g., EPO, hGH)
- Beta-2 agonists
- Hormone antagonists and modulators:
  - Aromatase inhibitors
  - Other estrogen receptor modulators (SERMS) and anti-estrogens
  - Agents modifying myostatin functions
- Diuretics and other masking agents (and related substances):
  - Diuretics
  - Masking agents
  - Plasma expanders

METHODS PROHIBITED IN AND OUT OF COMPETITION
- Enhancement of oxygen transfer:
  - Blood doping
  - Oxygen Transport
- Chemical and physical manipulation
- Gene doping

CLASSES OF SUBSTANCES PROHIBITED IN COMPETITION ONLY
- Stimulants (including D- and L-isomers where relevant)
- Narcotics
- Cannabinoids
- Glucocorticosteroids
- Alcohol
- Beta-blockers

SUBSTANCES PROHIBITED IN PARTICULAR SPORTS

■ **Alcohol: Prohibited in competition only:**
- Aeronautics (FAI) - (0.20 g/L)
- Archery (FITA, IPC) - (0.10 g/L)
- Automobile (FIA) - (0.10 g/L)
- Billiards (WCBS) - (0.20 g/L)
- Boules (CMSB) - (0.10 g/L)
- Disciplines involving shooting - (0.10 g/L)
- Karate (WKF) - (0.10 g/L)
- Modern Pentathlon (UIPM) - (0.10 g/L)
- Motorcycling (UIM) - (0.10 g/L)
- Powerboating (UIM) - (0.30 g/L)

■ **Beta-Blockers: Prohibited in-competition only:**
- Aeronautic (FAI)
- Archery (FITA, IPC)
- Automobile (FIA)
- Billiards (WCBS)
- Bobsleigh (FIBT) - freestyle aerials/halfpipe and snowboard
- Boules (CMSB, IPC bowls) - half-pipe or big air
- Bridge (FMB)
- Chess (FIDE)
- Curling (WCF)
- Gymnastics (FIG)
- Modern pentathlon (UIPM) for shooting
- Motorcycling (FIM)
- Nine-pin bowling (FIQ)
- Sailing (ISAF) for match race helms only (also prohibited out-of- of competition)
- Shooting (ISSF, IPC) (also prohibited out -of competition)
- Skiing/snowboarding (FIS) in ski jumping,
- Wrestling (FILA)

ERGOGENIC AIDS

- **Definition:** Substance designed to increase work or improve performance above that from regular training and diet.
  - Mechanical aids (e.g., running shoes).
  - Physiologic aids (e.g., fluids, blood).
  - Pharmacologic aids (e.g., amphetamines).
  - Nutritional aids (e.g., creatine, vitamins).

DIETARY SUPPLEMENTS

- **Definition:** Pills, powders, drinks, bars advertised to improve performance.
  - There is a lack of research or proof of effectiveness in the majority of products.
  - Lack of regulation and safety—supplements are not subject to FDA regulations.
  - Most athletes can meet their nutritional needs by consuming a well-balanced diet.
  - NCAA athletes should understand that most supplements are not regulated and may contain banned substances not listed on the label that may hurt their eligibility.
- **Commonly used dietary supplements:** Amino acids, bicarbonate, caffeine, creatine, coenzyme Q10, ephedrine (Ma Huang), ginseng, glucosamine, glutamine, glycerol, vitamins and minerals, antioxidants, protein supplements.

REVIEW OF SELECTED DRUGS AND SUPPLEMENTS

■ Amphetamines
- **Definition:** Stimulants sometimes used to treat obesity and attention deficit disorder.
- **Effects:** May improve strength, power, endurance, and time to exhaustion. Side effects include death from MI, CVA, and heat stroke. Other complications include, seizures, HTN, and arrhythmias. These are potentially addicting with chronic use.
- **Drug Testing:** Banned by the IOC and the NCAA.

■ Anabolic Steroids
- **Definition:** Anabolic-androgenic steroids (AAS): synthetic hormones that are analogues of testosterone.
- **Effects:** Androgenic (masculinizing) and anabolic (tissue building).
  - Administered PO, IM, or transdermally. Athletes may use numerous drugs with varying routes of administration or alternate routes over time.
    - Stacking: Using various routes simultaneously;
    - Cycling: Varying use pattern off and on several times per year.
  - Potential adverse effects on endocrine, GI, CV, MS, dermatologic, psychiatric, immunologic, and hematologic systems.
- **Drug Testing:** Banned by the IOC and NCAA.
NOTE: Metabolites of lipid-based drugs can be detected in urine for months vs. water-based injectables that can be detected for days or weeks.

■ Blood Doping and Erythropoietin (EPO)
- **Definition:** Artificially increases RBC mass to improve performance through infusion of RBCs or stimulating production with recombinant EPO (rEPO) thereby increasing O_2 carrying capacity.

- **Effects:** Increasing O_2 carrying capacity leads to increased aerobic power and aerobic capacity and increased time to exhaustion. Adverse effects include increased viscosity leading to thrombosis, stroke, or MI.
- **Drug Testing:** Banned by the IOC and NCAA and USADA. Transfusions from homologous blood can be detected. rEPO is still difficult to detect with current technology.

■ **Creatine (CK)**
- **Definition:** also known as phosphocreatine or creatine phosphokinase (CK); enzyme found in tissues, especially skeletal muscle; used for rapid regeneration of ATP.
- **Effects:** used to decrease workout recovery time; improve muscle strength and athletic performance. Studies show increases in repetitive strength tasks of short duration. Side effects include GI upset, muscle cramping. Safety in pediatric athletes is unclear.
- **Drug Testing:** Not a banned substance but the NCAA prohibits universities from providing it for their athletes.

■ **Caffeine**
- **Definition:** Mild stimulant found in drinks and other products.
- **Effects:** Enhanced performance during endurance events and shorter intense activity. Side effects include palpitations, insomnia, restlessness, and diarrhea. It does not appear to have any effects to increase risk for heat-related illness.
- **Drug Testing:** IOC limits urinary levels to 12 mcg/mL. NCAA allows 15 mcg/mL.

■ **Growth Hormone (GH)**
- **Definition:** Recombinant DNA techniques used to make synthetic form which is difficult to detect with current drug testing techniques.
- **Effects:** Anabolic effect; stimulation of skeletal muscle protein and nucleic acid; increase in lipolysis; enhanced healing after muscle injury. Increased improvement in performance is inconclusive. High HG levels are known to cause acromegaly. Long-term safety is unknown.
- **Drug Testing:** Banned by the IOC and NCAA. No current way to effectively test.

X ■ THE MEDICAL BAG

A team physician's medical bag is a collection of medical supplies necessary for sideline management. The contents of the bag should include items necessary for treating cardiac, orthopedic, pulmonary, ENT, musculoskeletal, and genitourinary emergencies that could arise during game coverage. Different sporting events will require different supplies; bag contents should be adjusted based upon location, weather conditions, and number of participants.

Due to limited space, the bag should contain frequently used medications or equipment that pertains to the activity. The American Medical Society for Sports Medicine has published a sideline preparedness consensus statement of medical bag supplies and also sideline supplies that may be useful.

GENERAL

Airway (oral and nasal)
Alcohol swabs
Antibiotics (topical and oral)
Antihistamines
Bandage scissors
Bandages (sterile, non-sterile, band-aids)
BP Cuff
Cricothyrotomy kit
Communication device (cell phone or other)
D-50W
Dental kit with solution for tooth storage
Disinfectant
Epi-pen
Eye kit with eye patches, blue light, fluorescein stain strips, ocular anesthetic, contact lens remover
Flashlight
Gloves (sterile and non-sterile)
Large bore angiocath
Local anesthetic/syringes/needles
Mouth-to-mouth mask
NSAID medications
Paper
Pen
Reflex hammer
Sharps box/container
Short acting beta-agonist inhaler
Stethoscope
Suture set or Steri-Strips
Wound irrigation materials

ALSO RECOMMENDED

ACLS supplies (including AED if needed and medications)
Cervical collar
Extremity splint material
Face mask removal tool
Ice
IV fluid and administration set
Nasal packing materials (tampons or nasal packing kits, decongestant nasal spray)
Ophthalmoscope
Oral fluid replacement
Otoscope
Oxygen with masks
Pulse oximeter
Rx pad
Sling
Spine board with attachments
Thermometer

XI ■ MISCELLANEOUS TOPICS

GENERAL NUTRITION FOR ATHLETES

- **Calories:** Amount of digestively available energy in food.
  - Average endurance athlete should consume approximately 55 kcal/kg body weight. Energy needs per day for strength training range from 33 to 60 kcal/kg for males and 30 to 44 kcal/kg for females.
- **Protein:** Organic compounds made of amino acids; it is the building block of muscle, bones, cartilage, enzymes, hormones.
  - RDA for sedentary individuals is 0.8 gm/kg body weight/day.
  - Male endurance athletes intake from 1.0 to 1.6 g/kg body weight/day or 150% to 175% of current RDA for protein.
  - Strength athletes intake 1.4 to 1.8g/kg body weight/day. Intakes >2 g/kg body weight/ day not shown to enhance muscle mass or performance.
  - Female athletes may require 10% to 20% less than males.
  - No increased protein requirement for athletes engaged in moderate-intensity endurance exercise.
  - Animal proteins are of higher quality than plant proteins, providing all essential amino acids for production of body proteins; plant proteins are not digested as well.
  - Animal proteins: meat, eggs, dairy products.
  - Plant proteins: grains, legumes, vegetables. Soy protein is a higher quality plant protein than other plant sources.
- **Carbohydrates (CHO):** Primary fuel used during exercise. Limited stores in body.
  - When depleted, athlete will feel fatigued.
  - Body converts CHO to muscle glycogen, one source of energy used by muscle.
  - General guidelines:
    - Nonendurance athletes 5 g/kg of body weight/day.
    - Endurance athletes are between 60% and 70% of total calories, or 8 to 10 g/kg body weight should be in the form of CHO for endurance events lasting longer than 1 hour or 6 g/kg body weight for endurance training for <1 hour/day.
- **Fats:** Storage form of energy in the body. As the duration of exercise increases, the relative utilization of fat increases.
  - Dietary fat should provide no more than 30% of total kilocalories per day. Endurance athletes can decrease intake to 20% to 25% to allow more carbohydrates.

SPORTS DRINKS AND HYDRATION RECOMMENDATIONS

FLUIDS AND HYDRATION IN SPORTS PEARLS

- Dehydration (of 2% or more) can reduce physical performance.
- Effects on performance may be most evident during exercise of duration greater than 1 hour or in environmental extremes.
- Water loss during exercise occurs primarily through sweat.
- Sweat rate is influenced by ambient temperature, humidity, exercise intensity, and rate of exogenous fluid intake.
- Dehydration → impaired heat dissipation → decreased plasma blood flow → decreased stroke volume → increased HR → cardiac compromise → heat stroke.
- Fluids should be consumed at a rate equal to the sweat rate.
- Fluid intake prior to exercise is necessary to offset risk of dehydration during exercise; fluid consumption of 400 to 600 mL 2 hours prior to activity is recommended.
- Fluid intake during exercise should equal fluid losses with a practical recommendation to consume 150 to 350 mL of water every 15 to 20 minutes.
- If activity is <1 hour, water only is recommended.
- If activity is >1 hour, addition of 4% to 8% carbohydrate and electrolyte can be beneficial.
- Optimal levels of carbohydrate and electrolyte promote better absorption, palatability and gastric emptying.
- Replace losses after activity with body weight changes being one method of determining fluid replacement amounts after exercise: 500 mL should be consumed for every 1 lb of weight loss.

ACSM AND NATA RECOMMENDATIONS:

- Drink 400 to 600mL (17 to 20 oz) of fluid 2 to 3 hours before exercise; another 7 to 10 oz, 10 to 20 minutes before an event, and then 150 to 350 mL (6 to 12 oz) every 15 to 20 minutes during exercise, beginning at the start of the activity.
- Following training or competition, it is necessary to rehydrate with 150% of fluid loss to completely rehydrate.
- Drink water with electrolytes and carbohydrates immediately after exercise if longer than 45 minutes or if intense.
- At equal intensity, requirements for fluid replacement becomes greater with increased sweating during environmental thermal stress.
- Check hydration status with body weight, urine color, and specific gravity.

SPORTS DRINKS PEARLS

- Optimal levels of Na+ and CHO stimulate the rate of fluid absorption and exhibit higher rates of gastric emptying compared to water.
- Improved taste can increase consumption compared to water.
- Sodium stimulates fluid absorption and helps the body "hold on" to fluid.
- Caffeinated beverages may improve endurance.

■ Optimal fluid replacement beverage contains:

CHO 4% to 8% (or 14 g per 8 oz); Na+ (10 to 20 mmol/L or 100 to 110 mg per 8 oz); K+ (3 to 5 mmol/L)

- Fructose-flavored beverages are absorbed slower compared to glucose, and sucrose and may contribute to GI distress.
- Carbonated beverages and fruit juices are not optimal because carbohydrate content is too high with low electrolyte content.
- Excessive fluid consumption can result in hyponatremia.

XII ■ CONSENSUS STATEMENTS AND POSITION STANDS

CONSENSUS STATEMENTS

The **American Medical Society for Sports Medicine** (www.amssm.org) and the **American College of Sports Medicine** (www.acsm.org) along with other organizations (American Academy of Family Physicians, American Academy of Orthopaedic surgeons, American Orthopaedic Society for Sports Medicine and the American Osteopathic Academy of Sports Medicine) have published "Consensus Statements" regarding different topics in Sports Medicine. The following is a list and brief synopses.

TEAM PHYSICIAN CONSENSUS STATEMENT (1999)

The objectives of the Team Physician Consensus Statement are to provide those individuals who are making decisions regarding medical care of athletes and teams a description of the duties of the team physician and a guideline regarding the qualifications of an adequately trained team physician. The purpose of this statement is to establish the importance of a qualified team physician to the decision makers so that the medical care of athletes is of the highest quality.

THE TEAM PHYSICIAN AND CONDITIONING OF ATHLETES FOR SPORTS: A CONSENSUS STATEMENT (2000)

This consensus statement discusses the fitness and conditioning principles regarding to sports participation. Specifically, strength training, aerobic conditioning, sports- specific conditioning, as well as specific recommendations for female, youth, and physically challenged athletes are discussed.

SIDELINE PREPAREDNESS FOR THE TEAM PHYSICIAN: A CONSENSUS STATEMENT (2001)

The objective of the Sideline Preparedness Consensus Statement is to educate physicians who provide practice or event coverage concise and specific recommendations regarding pre-season, game day, and post-season management. Medical and administrative protocols, as well as medical supplies for specific injuries, are presented.

RETURN TO PLAY ISSUES: A CONSENSUS STATEMENT (2002)

After evaluating injured or ill athletes, the team physician is faced with the responsibility to determine RTP criteria. This consensus statement is designed to assist the team physician to establish a return-to-play process.

FEMALE ATHLETE ISSUES FOR THE TEAM PHYSICIAN: A CONSENSUS STATEMENT (2003)

The goal of this section is to provide the team physician with knowledge specific to the care of the female athlete. Selected musculoskeletal and medical conditions are presented, along with epidemiologic considerations and essential and desirable objectives for the team physician to understand and to treat these conditions appropriately.

MASS PARTICIPATION EVENT MANAGEMENT FOR THE TEAM PHYSICIAN: A CONSENSUS STATEMENT (2004)

The team physician should be familiar with the principles unique to covering events where there are large numbers of participants. Varying environmental conditions, mixed age groups with varying athletic ability, along with anticipating injuries or illness and developing emergency action plans are presented

TEAM PHYSICIAN CONSENSUS STATEMENT—CONCUSSION (MILD TRAUMATIC BRAIN INJURY) (2005)

The purpose of the Team Physician Consensus Statement—Concussion (Mild Traumatic Brain Injury) is to define the common features of a concussion or mild traumatic brain injury (MTBI) and to assist the team physician with guidelines to provide optimal medical care of the athlete who suffers a MTBI.

PSYCHOLOGICAL ISSUES RELATED TO INJURY IN ATHLETES AND THE TEAM PHYSICIAN: A CONSENSUS STATEMENT (2006)

The goal of this consensus statement is to assist the team physician in relationship to psychologic issues related and accompanying athletic injury, injury rehabilitation and RTP. A section regarding principles regarding referring athletes to mental health providers is also presented.

SELECTED ISSUES IN INJURY AND ILLNESS PREVENTION AND THE TEAM PHYSICIAN: A CONSENSUS STATEMENT (2007)

Specific musculoskeletal injuries to the ankle, knee, and shoulder, head and neck injuries, cardiac illness, heat related illness, skin issues, and equipment issues are presented in this consensus statement. These conditions comprise many of the injuries or illnesses that the team physician will see in athletes.

HIV AND OTHER BLOOD-BORNE PATHOGENS IN SPORTS POSITION STATEMENT

This position statement discusses HIV and jepatitis B and C epidemiology and transmission. It specifically discusses management and preventative measures for sports events and participation. Finally, legal ramifications regarding blood-borne pathogens and sports participation are discussed.

MONONUCLEOSIS AND ATHLETIC PARTICIPATION: AN EVIDENCED-BASED SUBJECT REVIEW (2008)

The clinical presentation of infectious mononucleosis and its management in regard to athletic participation is the subject of this position statement.

POSITION STANDS

The American College has several position stands that are based upon solid research and scientific data. These are available at www.acsm-msse.org. They include the following:

- **October 1, 2007:** The Female Athlete Triad
- **May 1, 2007:** Exercise and Acute Cardiovascular Events: Placing the Risks into Perspective
- **March 1, 2007:** Exertional Heat Illness during Training and Competition
- **February 1, 2007:** Exercise and Fluid Replacement.
- **November 1, 2006:** Prevention of Cold Injuries during Exercise.
- **November 1, 2004:** Physical Activity & Bone Health
- **March 1, 2004:** Exercise & Hypertension
- **March 1, 2002:** AEDs in Health/Fitness Facilities
- **February 1, 2002:** Progression Models in Resistance Training for Healthy Adults
- **December 1, 2001:** Appropriate Intervention Strategies for Weight Loss and Prevention of Weight Regain for Adults
- **December 1, 2000:** Nutrition and Athletic Performance
- **July 1, 2000:** Exercise and Type 2 Diabetes
- **June 1, 1998:** The Recommended Quantity and Quality of Exercise for Developing and Maintaining Cardiorespiratory and Muscular Fitness, and Flexibility in Healthy Adults Exercise and Physical Activity for Older Adults AHA/ACSM Joint Statement: Recommendations for Cardiovascular Screening, Staffing, and Emergency Policies at Health/Fitness Facilities
- **December 1, 1997:** ADA/ACSM Joint Statement: Diabetes Mellitus Exercise
- **June 1, 1996:** The Use of Blood Doping as an Ergogenic Aid Weight Loss in Wrestlers
- **March 1, 1994:** Exercise for Patients with Coronary Artery Disease
- **May 1, 1987:** The Use of Anabolic-Androgenic Steroids in Sports
- **June 1, 1982:** The Use of Alcohol in Sports

XIII ■ EXERCISE PHYSIOLOGY

BASIC EXERCISE PHYSIOLOGY

- **Definition:** branch of physiology discipline that focuses on the integration of physiological functions that enable exercise
- **Muscle action:**
  - Concentric: contract or shorten
  - Eccentric: lengthen or extend
  - Isometric/static: remain the same length
- **Lactic Acid (LA):** Provides fuel source to working muscles, not a useless metabolic byproduct of muscle metabolism.
  - Its role in muscle soreness has been disproved.
  - LA is a key substance used to provide energy, produce liver glycogen and blood glucose. 65% of lactic acid is converted to CO_2 and water, 20% into glycogen, 10% into protein, and 5% into glucose.
  - Lactate: product of glycolysis.
  - Formed from pyruvate (during exercise) in recycling of NAD or when insufficient O_2 is available for pyruvate to enter the TCA cycle. Resynthesized by the liver (Cori cycle) to form glucose.
  - Extent of lactate formation depends on availability of both pyruvate and NADH. If the lactate threshold is reached during exercise, excessive LA can accumulate and cause fatigue. This can be offset by proper training and high CHO diet.
  - Blood lactate at rest: 0.8 to 1.5 mM
  - During exercise: in excess of 18 mM

OXYGEN UPTAKE (VO_2)

$VO_2 = CO \times (a-VOs) = HR \times SV \times (a-VO_2)$
Average adult at rest: 5 L/min and during strenuous exercise: 20 to 30 L/min

MAXIMAL HR

Highest HR achieved during standardized maximal exercise testing.
Two formulas used: Max HR = 220 – age or 208 – 0.7 x age.

HR RESERVE (HRR)

Difference between max HR during max exercise testing and resting HR.
Smaller difference, the lower the reserve and the narrower the range for exercise.

TARGET TRAINING HR

Karvonen Formula: Use 50% and 85% of HRR:
0.50 x HRR + Resting HR and 0.85 x HRR + Resting HR

METABOLIC ENERGY EQUIVALENT (MET)

Energy cost of activities in terms of multiples of resting metabolic rate. Used by CDC to recommend exercise intensity.
- 1 to 3 MET: Eating, dressing, walking around house.
- 4 to 10 MET: Climbing flight of stairs, walking on level ground, playing a game of golf.
- 10 MET: Strenuous sports; swimming, singles tennis, football.

BORG SCALE OR RATING OF PERCEIVED EXERTION (RPE)

Scale for an individual to rate "degree of physical strain."

PHYSIOLOGIC CHANGES IN THE GERIATRIC ATHLETE

Cardiovascular function:
- VO_2 max ↓5% to 15% per decade after age 25 years
- HR max ↓ 6 to 10 BPM per decade
- ↓ Plasma, red cell, total blood volume
- ↓ Ejection fraction and LV contractility
- ↓ CV response to submaximal exercise
- Higher BP response
- ↓ Total muscle mass ~50% between ages 20 and 90 years old
- Strength declines ~15% per decade in 6th and 7th decades and >30% thereafter

PRINCIPLES OF EXERCISE TRAINING

- **FITT:** Frequency, Intensity, Time (duration), Type of exercise.
- **Overload:** Gains in strength/endurance come when greater demands are placed on the cardiopulmonary and musculoskeletal system.
- **Periodization:** Altering training variables to achieve gains.
- **Phases:** Getting body ready for new activity: 4 weeks; strength development: 4 to 7 weeks; muscular endurance: 8 to 12 weeks.

■ Plyometrics
- **Definition:** Method of training for power or explosiveness that involves jumping, bounding, and hopping. Specifically focused on rapid pairing of eccentric and concentric contractions, or stretch/shortening cycles to produce increased power.

  Force generated by lengthening contraction (eccentric) can be markedly increased if it is followed by a shortening contraction (concentric).

EXERCISE PHYSIOLOGY AND THE SYSTEMS

■ **Gastrointestinal System**
  • Initial exercise: 15% of splanchnic blood flow shunted during exercise.
  • As core temp increases, 20% is shunted to the skin for temp regulation and cooling.
  • Maximum exercise: 80% splanchnic blood flow is shunted.
  • Gastric emptying time (GET): Increases as exercise begins and level reaches 75% of VO2 max then decreases. Emotional stress can slow GET and lead to vomiting.
  • Rapid accumulation of lactic acid or culmination of endurance events may cause vomiting.
  • Gastroesophageal reflux: Related to air swallowing and lower esophageal sphincter relaxation in exercise.

■ **Renal Function**
  • Renal perfusion decreases as adrenaline and noradrenalin activate the sympathetic nervous system and cause vasoconstriction.
  • Strenuous exercise can decrease renal blood flow by 75%
  • Proteinuria found in up to 70% to 80% of athletes but must investigate if persists.
  • Increased hematuria with increased duration and intensity of activity; usually resolves within 48 to 72 hours.
  • Repeat after resting for 72 hours. If positive on 2 or more of 3 samples, must investigate.
  • Microtrauma: Empty bladder contused as posterior wall hits the fixed trigone and/or increased permeability of glomerulus.

INDEX

T

NOTES